Despite headline-making news, the average American still consumes only about half the recommended amount of folic acid and other B vitamins daily. But consider the following:

• In 1998, the U.S. Food and Drug Administration ordered that folic acid—a member of the vitamin B family—be added to all wheat products, most breakfast cereals, bread, fortified rice, and pasta.

• In 1998, the prestigious Cleveland Clinic revealed that low levels of $B_6$ and folic acid can increase the risk of heart disease and stroke.

• In 1992, the U.S. Public Health Service recommended that all women of childbearing age consume 400 micrograms of folic acid daily to reduce the risk of birth defects.

• Studies show that depressed patients consistently have low blood levels of folic acid, and the greater the deficiency, the worse the depression. One theory is that the body needs folic acid to manufacture the chemicals that transmit messages throughout the brain and body.

• Lack of $B_{12}$, the vitamin necessary for the formation of red blood cells, energy, and growth may lead to anemia and fatigue, vulnerability to infection, bruising, and nerve disorders. In turn, vitamin $B_6$ is required for the proper absorption of $B_{12}$ and magnesium and in aiding insomnia, irritability, and depression.

# Folic Acid and the Amazing B Vitamins

## A Question-and-Answer Guide for Women and Men

Glenn S. Rothfeld, M.D., M.Ac.,
& Suzanne LeVert

BERKLEY BOOKS, NEW YORK

FOLIC ACID AND THE AMAZING B VITAMINS

A Berkley Book / published by arrangement with
the authors

PRINTING HISTORY
Berkley edition / March 2000

The Penguin Putnam Inc. World Wide Web site address is
http://www.penguinputnam.com

ISBN: 0-425-17369-0

BERKLEY®
Berkley Books are published by The Berkley Publishing Group,
a division of Penguin Putnam Inc., 375 Hudson Street,
New York, New York 10014.
BERKLEY and the ''B'' design
are trademarks belonging to Penguin Putnam Inc.

PRINTED IN THE UNITED STATES OF AMERICA

10  9  8  7  6  5  4  3

# Contents

# · 1 ·

# Understanding the Power of the Bs

Heart disease, the leading cause of death in the United States today. Birth defects, a heartbreaking reality for thousands of families every year. Cancer, a painful, often deadly disease that strikes old and young alike in sobering numbers. And then there are some less serious but nonetheless troublesome ailments that plague millions: insomnia, mood swings, fatigue, muscle and joint pain, bleeding and sore gums, and problems with concentration.

Seems like a rather disparate list of illnesses and complaints, doesn't it? Well, as we'll show you throughout this book, all of them—and a host of others—have at least one common element: They can develop because the body does not receive enough of a particular group of chemicals called B vitamins. Indeed, without these substances in sufficient quantities, the body virtually breaks down, its cells unable to perform their functions properly.

The good news is that the reverse is equally true, that by providing your body with enough of the B vitamins, you dramatically increase your chances of staving off illness in the future and improving the way you feel every day. Before we get to the prescriptive elements, however, we want you to understand what vitamins are and how they work in the body.

## THE VITAMIN STORY

When you think about vitamins—and their nutrient counterparts, minerals—it may help to imagine your body as an enormous chemical lab, with each cell of the body performing a series of conversions and processes that together sustain life. In order to keep the body up and running, the cells require a number of different substances, including vitamins and minerals to perform their intricate work. In essence, vitamins and minerals act as catalysts in the chemical reactions taking place in our bodies. Again, if just one of those substances is not present in sufficient quantities, disease and dysfunction may develop.

Today, research indicates that people can have mild or moderate vitamin deficiencies that arise for a variety of reasons. Although these deficiencies may not cause immediate or obvious diseases, they can affect your health in profound ways today and in the future. We'll discuss this concept in more depth, especially as it relates to the B vitamins. For now, let's explore the world of vitamins and how they work in the body.

### What exactly is a vitamin?

A vitamin is a nutrient, which is a substance obtained from food and used by the body for growth, maintenance, or repair of tissues. There are six categories of nutrients:

water, protein, carbohydrates, fat, vitamins, and minerals. With a few exceptions, the body cannot manufacture the chemicals it derives from these nutrients, which means that most of them come from our food or from supplements.

Nutrients function in one or more of three general ways: They furnish the body with heat and energy, they provide material for growth and repair of body tissues, and they assist in the regulation of body processes. Vitamins help regulate the conversion of food to energy in the body. Some vitamins—like the B vitamins—primarily work to help the body convert food into energy. The B vitamins activate specific metabolic facilitators called enzymes, which control digestion and the absorption and use of proteins, fats, and carbohydrates.

Vitamins are divided into two categories: water-soluble vitamins and fat-soluble vitamins. The water-soluble vitamins are the B vitamins and vitamin C. Your body uses water-soluble vitamins quickly—as soon as the digestive system absorbs them—and whatever the body fails to use, it excretes into the urine within three to four days. That's why, as you'll see, it is extremely difficult to consume toxic levels of these vitamins. Fat-soluble vitamins, on the other hand, are stored in fat and organ tissue, particularly the liver. You have to be much more careful about using appropriate amounts of the fat-soluble vitamins A, D, E, and K because you can build up excess, toxic levels if you consume too much of one or more of these vitamins.

### How does the body use vitamins?

The body generally doesn't use vitamins as they occur in food but instead must first transform them into simpler forms called coenzymes or cofactors. For example, when you eat a piece of liver, your body first must convert raw material from a protein (called tryptophan) into the active forms of niacin called nicotinamide adenine dinucleotide (NAD) or nicotinamide adenine dinucleotide phosphate (NADP). These substances are the ones that do the real work, metabolically speaking. Interestingly, this conversion process often requires the presence of other vitamins and minerals in their active forms in order to take place. For the body to convert tryptophan into the active forms of niacin, for example, you need vitamin $B_6$, riboflavin (another B vitamin), and iron.

Needless to say, you don't need to understand the highly complicated (but fascinating) chemical processes your body performs on the food you eat in order to provide your cells with the substances they need to function. But it is awesome to consider just what goes on under the skin, so to speak, as you go about your daily business. It's also important to be aware that the food you eat is not simply a source of pleasure and satiety: It provides the raw materials you need to stay healthy and active.

## Do we get all the vitamins we need from our food?

In a perfect world, the best source of vitamins and minerals would be a healthy, balanced diet of fresh foods and lean proteins. That's because fresh, whole food contains a variety of vitamins and minerals that scientists believe act together in very special ways and in specific combinations—ways and combinations that apparently can't be reproduced in a multivitamin supplement. The truth is, as advanced as science has become, it still can neither completely understand nor perfectly duplicate the way Mother Nature works.

Unfortunately, a healthy, balanced diet eludes most

Americans as they head into the twenty-first century, and for three reasons. First and most commonly, we just don't eat the right kinds of foods in the right amounts. In chapter 3, we'll explore the world of the Food Guide Pyramid, the one that most nutritional experts recommend, which emphasizes complex carbohydrates (like whole-grain breads and brown rice), fresh fruits and vegetables, and lean protein, rather than processed foods, fat, and sugar.

Second, even if we ate all the right foods in the right amounts, we might not get enough of the nutrients we need because the modern world of food production robs fruits and vegetables of much of their natural vitamin and mineral content. The soil in which we grow food tends to be less rich in nutrients than in the past, and chemical fertilizers further erode soil integrity. In addition, fruits and vegetables are frequently shipped from great distances, aging along the way and thus losing some of their nutritional value as a result. To make matters worse, cooking vegetables, legumes, and fruits also depletes them of their nutritional value.

Third, our bodies are not able to absorb all the nutrients contained in the food we eat. For example, according to Dr. Jesse F. Gregory II, professor of food science and human nutrition at the University of Florida in Gainesville, we absorb perhaps no more than 50 percent of the folic acid that occurs naturally in food. That means that although a cup of lentils may contain almost 400 micrograms of folic acid, our bodies can only absorb and use 200 micrograms.

All this goes to show you that, in addition to eating a healthy, balanced diet, you should consider taking vitamin supplements. We'll discuss that at more length in chapter 2 and elsewhere, but it is an important point to keep in mind.

**What happens when we don't obtain all the vitamins and minerals our bodies need to function?**

If a vitamin or mineral deficiency is severe enough, overt disease will occur. For instance, a profound lack of vitamin C causes the disease scurvy, which has symptoms involving wounds that don't heal, muscle pain, bleeding gums, fatigue, and pneumonia. If untreated, scurvy can be fatal. A severe deficiency of vitamin $B_3$, or niacin, results in a disease called pellagra, which causes a wide range of disabling, debilitating symptoms including neurological damage, severe skin disease, and gastrointestinal disorders.

In modern, industrial nations like the United States, overt vitamin deficiencies are rare, although they do occur in certain populations such as the drug- and alcohol-addicted, the very poor, and the neglected elderly. However, increasing scientific evidence indicates that even marginal, relatively mild deficiencies can interfere with the quality and length of life.

**What else can cause vitamin and mineral deficiencies?**

In addition to a poor diet, several other factors can affect your vitamin and mineral status. These factors include alcohol use and abuse; use of prescription and over-the-counter medications; certain chronic and acute illnesses; and chronic stress. Each of these conditions makes it more difficult for you to obtain all the nutrients you need to survive and thrive, and here's why:

• *Decrease in appetite.* Taking medication, feeling ill or under stress, or abusing alcohol all limit your appetite, making it less likely that you'll consume enough of the right kinds of food to meet your nutritional needs.

• *Interference with nutrient absorption or use.* Alcohol and medications can bind themselves to nutrients and change, tamper with digestive juices and enzymes that break down nutrients, and/or increase excretion of nutrients—all of which prevent the body from being able to use them efficiently.

• *Irritation of the digestive tract.* By irritating the digestive tract, alcohol and certain medications can inhibit the absorption of folic acid, protein, calcium, and vitamins $B_1$, $B_{12}$, A, D, and E.

• *Destruction of nutrients.* Inhaling tobacco removes vitamin C from the tissues and lowers absorption of vitamins $B_6$, A, and beta-carotene.

When it comes to the B vitamins, we'll get more specific about which medications and lifestyle choices will interfere most with their absorption and use later in the book. For now, it's important to understand that—even if you are one of the relatively few Americans who eat a balanced, healthy diet every day—you may still run the risk of having a marginal vitamin deficiency and therefore could benefit from taking one or more nutritional supplements.

**This book is all about B vitamins. Are they more important than other nutrients?**

Not at all. As discussed, your body requires a range of vitamins and minerals that all work together, in marvelous combinations that science has yet to fully understand. Taking only B vitamins, or just one of the B vitamins, in higher than usual amounts can lead to metabolic imbalances that cause unpleasant symptoms and even serious disease. What we're trying to stress in this book is that because of our modern lifestyle, we may not be getting enough of *all* of the vitamins and minerals we need, and of particular interest and importance in this discussion are the B vitamins, which serve to promote health in unique and essential ways. Let's take a look.

## UNDERSTANDING THE B VITAMINS

A group of eight closely related nutrients, the B vitamins play many crucial roles in the body. Working together as a team, these vitamins work to create and maintain DNA (the genetic code that directs the growth and function of every cell in the body); support the health of the skin, hair, and nails; help metabolize carbohydrate, fat, and protein for energy; and participate in the proper function of the brain and nervous system. Although overt B vitamin deficiencies are rare, more and more evidence is mounting that even a mild deficiency of one or more of these essential nutrients leaves the body open to disease. As you'll see, vitamin B deficiencies are linked to a wide range of conditions, including heart disease and stroke, cancer, Alzheimer's disease and mood disorders, and debilitating skin and joint conditions such as psoriasis and rheumatoid arthritis.

**It seems that every other day we're hearing about another miracle vitamin or another miracle cure for just about every ailment under the sun. For a while, it was vitamin C, then it was beta-carotene, and now it's folic acid and the other B vitamins. Is it possible for one substance to do it all?**

That's an excellent question that has one simple answer: Absolutely not. As we'll emphasize throughout this book, each nutrient is equally valuable and no single one is more important than another. Although scientific testing has allowed us to isolate the substances from food that are essential to health, so far, all the data suggest that the true power of vitamins and minerals comes from the special combinations they form within food. Taking folic acid—or any single vitamin, for that matter—in total isolation will, in fact, only result in putting you at risk for serious disease and dysfunction. We'll show you as we go along the importance of balancing your diet and your vitamin supplement intake.

To be fair, however, much of the excitement you see in the media and among scientists is in large part honest enthusiasm and appreciation for a new understanding of the power of vitamins in preventing and healing disease. In recent years, scientists have revealed the importance of the B vitamins to the health of the heart, to a healthy pregnancy, and to the treatment of myriad diseases. That's good news indeed, because all it takes is eating a balanced diet and taking safe, effective, and inexpensive supplements.

## How many different kinds of B vitamins are there?

Scientists have isolated eight different substances that come under the broad heading of B vitamins. Although quite similar in many ways, each has a slightly different chemical makeup, is required by the body in varying amounts, and performs different though related functions. They include:

- Vitamin $B_1$, also known as thiamine

- Vitamin $B_2$, also known as riboflavin

- Vitamin $B_3$, also known as niacin and niacinamide

- Vitamin $B_5$, better known as pantothenic acid

- Vitamin $B_6$, or pyroxidine

- Vitamin $B_{12}$, or cobalamin

- Folic acid, or folate

- Biotin

In addition to these main substances, the B vitamins require several cofactors that work in harmony with the essential nutrients to aid in the breakdown and conversion of food into cellular energy and also help support all of the body's physical and mental functions. Vitamin B cofactors include choline, inositol, coenzyme Q-10, and lipoic acid. We'll be discussing these substances in the course of the book as well.

## I've heard of the B-complex vitamin. What is it?

Because the B vitamins and their cofactors work so closely with one another—in fact, a deficiency or excess of just one creates an imbalance in them all—scientists have created a supplement that combines all of these substances together in an appropriate mix, a mix that mirrors as much as possible the way they are found together in foods and in the body. Taking a B-complex supplement every day will allow you to increase the amount you take of another B vitamin for therapeutic reasons. If you're pregnant, for instance, and want to take extra folic acid, taking a B-complex supplement (or a good multivitamin with sufficient levels of B vitamins in it) will prevent you from developing an unhealthy imbalance or deficiency of another B vitamin. We'll discuss this at more length in chapter 2.

## How do the B vitamins affect our health?

One primary function of the B vitamins is to aid in the conversion of food—protein, carbohydrates, and fats—into glucose, the energy that cells need in order to function properly. Without sufficient B vitamins, your body doesn't get the fuel it needs, which is why one of the first symptoms of a B vitamin deficiency is fatigue. They also help to synthesize certain neurotransmitters (brain chemicals that help transmit messages throughout the nervous system) and fatty acids (substances necessary for the maintenance of nerve tissue as well as the health of the skin, hair, and nails). The B vitamins are also necessary for the formation of DNA, the genetic code that regulates the proper function of every cell in the body.

In addition, certain of the B vitamins serve two other primary functions in the body: They protect cells from becoming damaged, and they participate in a chemical reaction that lowers the level of a potentially toxic substance called homocysteine. Let's take a look.

- *The B vitamins as antioxidants.* Many of the B vitamins are known as antioxidants, substances that can protect cells from becoming damaged by toxins. This antioxidant effect helps reduce the risk of several potentially deadly and debilitating diseases, including cancer and heart disease. Most cancers, for instance, start with a mutation, or random change, to DNA—the genetic code found in each and every cell. The B vitamins—particularly riboflavin, $B_6$, $B_{12}$, pantothenic acid, and folic acid—are necessary to prevent this damage from occurring in the first place as well as to repair the damage once it occurs.

- *The B vitamins and homocysteine.* A body chemical

known as homocysteine has been implicated in a wide variety of diseases and conditions, including heart disease, Alzheimer's disease, osteoporosis, and certain birth defects, among others. One important function of several of the B vitamins is to reduce the level of this chemical in the blood. As you'll see in future chapters, the relationship between B vitamin intake, homocysteine levels, and health is a crucial and fascinating one, still under investigation by scientists and physicians around the world.

**I've heard about antioxidants and free radicals. What exactly are they and how do they affect health?**

Antioxidants are enzymes, vitamins, and minerals that mop up free radicals, which are molecules in the body that contain one or more unpaired electrons in their orbits. These unstable molecules destroy healthy cells in an attempt to stabilize themselves. This process damages healthy cells, sometimes beyond repair. Left to run rampant, free radicals can batter our proteins, cell membranes, and then reach the cell core of DNA. They can clog the walls of our arteries, kill brain cells, stiffen and deplete our muscles, and throw our immune systems out of kilter. The damage done to enzymes, cell membranes, and DNA may lead to the development of several serious conditions, including heart disease, Alzheimer's disease, cancer, arthritis, and others.

To protect itself against free radical damage, the human body requires antioxidants. We produce some antioxidants internally, others we ingest in the foods we eat. Antioxidants disarm free radicals in a variety of ways and then other body chemicals mop up the remnants of these once-harmful molecules before they can do any damage to the body. Among the most important antioxidants are the vitamins C, E, and beta-carotene (a precursor to vitamin A). However, more and more evidence indicates that other vitamins—including many of the B vitamins—also work to protect our cells from free radical damage, which is why it's so important to evaluate your intake and make adjustments if necessary. Doing so could help you maintain your health and feel more vital.

### What exactly is homocysteine? Where does it come from?

Homocysteine is a breakdown product of the amino acid methionine, a component of the protein we ingest in food. Methionine is one of the building blocks used by the body to manufacture its own proteins to use in building muscle, bone, and other tissue. In the normal course of metabolism, some of the methionine in the body breaks down to homocysteine, which is, in turn, converted either back to methionine or to other compounds, particularly a substance called cysteine.

The B vitamins—particularly vitamin $B_6$, folic acid, and vitamin $B_{12}$—are crucial to this conversion process. Without their presence, too much homocysteine can build up in the bloodstream, which, as discussed, can have toxic effects on several different body systems, most prominently the heart and blood vessels. In fact, the American Heart Association recently added elevated homocysteine levels to the risk factors for cardiovascular disease, placing it alongside high cholesterol, obesity, and diabetes as indicative of an increased risk of heart attack and stroke. There is also mounting evidence that homocysteine plays a role in the development of such diseases as Alzheimer's disease, osteoporosis, and rheumatoid arthritis.

## What specific diseases and conditions do the B vitamins affect?

You might be surprised at just how integral the B vitamins are to your everyday health as well as to the prevention and treatment of disease. In chapter 8 of this book, we'll outline how the B vitamins affect specific conditions, but here's a broad overview to get you started:

• *Birth defects.* The B vitamins, particularly folic acid and the coenzyme choline, play essential roles in the development of fetal brain and spinal cord tissue—such essential roles, in fact, that the Federal Food and Drug Administration required that folic acid be added to specific flour, breads, and other grains to help ensure that women of childbearing age get enough of this B vitamin. We'll discuss this connection in chapter 4.

• *Heart disease and stroke.* The role that the B vitamins play in reducing homocysteine levels is profound, and several studies now prove that link. For instance, according to a fourteen-year examination of 80,000 nurses called the Nurses' Health Study, women who ingested the largest amount of folic acid and $B_6$ faced about half the risk of heart disease, even after researchers adjusted for factors such as age, hypertension, smoking, fiber, and vitamin E intake. The National Institute of Neurological Disorders and Stroke of the National Institutes of Health is now investigating whether the nutrients would prevent second strokes or heart attacks in patients who have already had one mild, nondisabling stroke. You'll read more about the Bs and the cardiovascular system in chapter 5.

• *Cancer.* Because of the ability of the B vitamins to

protect cells from damage, their role in cancer prevention and treatment has been under investigation for decades. In particular, a connection has been made between cervical dysplasia—a precursor to cervical cancer in women—and B vitamin intake, and a 1998 study published in the *Annals of Internal Medicine* showed that using multivitamin supplements with folic acid for fifteen years or more may decrease the risk of colon cancer by about 75 percent. You'll find more on the results of these studies and others in chapter 6.

• *Nervous system and mood disorders.* The B vitamins have a long history as antistress nutrients and mood enhancers, primarily because they help produce brain chemicals called neurotransmitters. Deficiencies of these vitamins—and perhaps only mild deficiencies—could be related to depression, schizophrenia, and other mental disorders.

• *Skin, hair, and nail problems.* Among the first symptoms to develop when one or more of the B vitamins are deficient are skin disorders, which include flaking of the skin around the eyes and nose, brittle nails, and hair loss. That's partly because of the role the B vitamins play in DNA synthesis and maintenance; when a deficiency exists, the cells in the body that turn over the fastest—like skin cells—suffer the most damage. The role the Bs play in protein metabolism and synthesis is also important, since protein is an important component of these tissues.

• *Muscle and joint problems.* Current research suggest that the B vitamins—primarily vitamin $B_6$—can both stave off the development of and treat certain conditions that affect the muscles and joints and the nerves that feed them, such as carpal tunnel syndrome, arthritis, and bursitis.

• *Gastrointestinal disorders.* The relationship between B vitamins and gastrointestinal disorders like diarrhea, colitis, and Crohn's disease is one of both cause and effect. Malnutrition can cause wasting diarrhea and irritation of the digestive tract, and the loss of nutrients through diarrhea and malabsorption of nutrients that results can further deplete the B vitamins. In addition, folic acid and other B vitamins help to preserve the mucous membranes that line the digestive tract.

• *Stress-related problems.* Most illnesses are affected by stress. Vitamin $B_6$ and other B vitamins, as well as the mineral magnesium, are required by the adrenal gland to produce the hormones that control our stress response (including adrenaline and cortisol) as well as the sexual hormones.

In the chapters that follow, we'll explore the role of B vitamins in health and disease in further detail. For now, let's take a closer look at why you and your family may need to increase your intake of these vital nutrients.

## GETTING ENOUGH OF THE Bs

As discussed, most Americans don't get enough of all the B vitamins they need, mainly because our diets are known for their concentration on nutrient-poor fast foods. Not only do such diets fail to provide enough of the vitamins and minerals you need, but they also deplete the existing B vitamins more rapidly. In addition, cooking food may destroy the potency of several B vitamins.

## How can I tell if I'm deficient in B vitamins?

Mild vitamin B deficiencies, the kind that are more likely to affect most Americans, tend to have relatively subtle physical symptoms. Among the most obvious symptoms are those we term psychological—irritability, nervousness, and depression—but every part of the body can be affected. And the longer the deficiency lasts, the more damage can occur to the body.

In chapter 2, we outline for you the deficiency symptoms for each of the B vitamins in some detail. For now, here's a quick rundown of what you might expect:

• $B_1$ deficiency can cause tingling or loss of sensation in the legs, weakness, heart problems, mental changes, abdominal changes.

• $B_2$ deficiency results in cracked lips, pallor, and a sore tongue.

• Niacin deficiency can cause fatigue and weakness, poor appetite, inflamed skin, burning mouth and tongue, indigestion and nausea, and mental changes.

• $B_6$ deficiency can cause dermatitis, sore mouth and tongue, PMS, abdominal pain, diarrhea, and mental changes.

• $B_{12}$ deficiency can cause symptoms that range from pernicious anemia to fatigue and neuropathies.

• Folic acid deficiency can cause a decrease in the healing of mucous membrane tissues and can result in birth defects if the deficiency is in a pregnant woman.

## Where are B vitamins found in food?

In chapter 3, we'll give you a complete rundown of dietary sources and offer you some tips about creating a healthy eating plan that provides you with ample quantities of the B vitamins. All the B vitamins are found in brewer's yeast, liver, and whole-grain cereals. Other good sources of certain B vitamins include green leafy vegetables, eggs, dried beans, fish, poultry, lean meats, organ meats, and nuts. Under the National Food Fortification program, most foods made with processed flours also contain levels of thiamine, riboflavin, niacin, and folic acid.

## Is it possible to get all the B vitamins you need from a balanced diet?

It's perhaps possible, but only if you're a perfectly healthy person who eats primarily fresh vegetables and lean meat (preferably organ meat) cooked with care, who doesn't drink alcohol, smoke cigarettes, or live under stress, and who isn't pregnant. Otherwise, it's tough to get all you need from your diet. That's why most experts—even those in the mainstream medical community—now suggest supplementing your diet with the careful use of vitamin supplements.

## Are there any specific populations at special risk for vitamin B deficiency?

Groups particularly in need of higher B-vitamin intake include the elderly; women who are pregnant, lactating, or taking birth control pills (which are known to deplete the B vitamins); people on calorie-restricted diets or who are vegetarians (who may not consume enough high-quality B vitamins); smokers (because smoking depletes all vitamins and minerals, especially folic acid and $B_{12}$); and those whose diets are high in alcohol or caffeine (which contain tannin, a B vitamin–depleting substance). People who are under constant stress use up their B vitamins at a rapid rate. Also, people who consume a diet low in whole grains and vegetables and high in processed foods may need more B vitamins as food processing can destroy these nutrients.

In addition, people who suffer certain gastrointestinal conditions such as ulcerative colitis or disease-related diarrhea are prone to loss of the B vitamins. Some substances such as sulfa drugs, sleeping pills, insecticides, and estrogen (as found in birth control pills and estrogen replacement therapy) can create a condition in the digestive tract that can destroy these vitamins.

### I've heard that antibiotics also deplete vitamin B supplies. Is this true?

Yes, it is true. Antibiotics can kill beneficial bacteria that normally live in your large intestine and produce small amounts of some B vitamins. If you're taking certain antibiotics, then, you may become vitamin deficient. For that reason, some doctors recommend replacing the beneficial bacteria with acidophilus (the good bacteria), with supplements, or by eating lots of yogurt during and after antibiotic treatment. We'll discuss that recommendation further in relevant chapters.

### Are women at special risk for vitamin B deficiency?

Yes, they are. Women who plan to become pregnant need to pay special attention to their intake of folic acid because—as we'll discuss in depth in chapter 4—adequate levels of this vitamin are crucial to the proper development of the fetus early in the pregnancy. Furthermore, once pregnant, women need to boost their intake of all essential nutrients in order to provide the fetus with proper nutrition during gestation. If women breast-feed, they need to maintain this higher intake during this period.

Women who take birth control pills are also at risk for B vitamin deficiency—particularly of folic acid—since oral contraceptives are known to deplete folic acid and other nutrients. Premenstrual syndrome frequently responds to B vitamin supplementation, especially vitamin $B_6$. Furthermore, women who suffer from cervical dysplasia (the development of abnormal cells on the cervix) and who take birth control pills may benefit greatly from taking high doses of folic acid. We'll discuss this at more length in chapter 6.

Finally, after menopause, women have to pay special attention to the intake of the B vitamins. Before this stage of life, the hormone estrogen apparently protects women against the buildup of homocysteine and the damage this body chemical does to various tissues of the body. With the loss of estrogen at menopause, this protective factor disappears, setting the stage for the development of cardiovascular disease, osteoporosis, and other degenerative diseases related to the buildup of homocysteine. Having plentiful folic acid, $B_6$, and $B_{12}$ supplies on hand in the body can help mitigate these effects.

## Why are the elderly at high risk for B vitamin deficiency?

There are a variety of reasons why the elderly are at special risk for B vitamin deficiency. First, many seniors fail to eat a healthy diet. The reason for this failure include loss of appetite due to illness and/or difficulty chewing due to loss of teeth. Second, the digestive tract requires a substance called hydrochloric acid (HCl) to absorb vitamin $B_{12}$ and other nutrients. HCl stimulates a chemical called *intrinsic factor,* which is crucial to proper nutrient absorption. Unfortunately, HCl production naturally declines with age and is also affected by certain medications often ingested by the elderly, including the heavy use of acid-blocking drugs that is prevalent in that population. Finally, as a group, the elderly take more medications than other segments of the population, medications that interfere with the proper absorption and metabolism of nutrients of all kinds, especially of folic acid, vitamin $B_6$, and vitamin $B_{12}$.

Now that you've received a broad overview of the importance of the B vitamins and why you may be at risk for a deficiency, let's move on to a more specific discussion of each of these remarkable nutrients in chapter 2.

## REFERENCES FOR CHAPTER ONE

Joosten, E; Van den Berg, A; Reizler, R; et al. "More evidence that deficiencies of vitamin $B_{12}$, folate, and vitamin $B_6$ commonly occur in elderly people." *American Journal of Clinical Nutrition,* 1993; 58: 468–476.

Mayer, FL; Jacobsen, DW; Robinson, K. "Homocysteine and coronary atherosclerosis." *Journal of American College of Cardiology,* 1996; 27 (3): 517–527.

Swain, RA; St. Clair, L. "The role of folic acid in deficiency states and prevention of disease." *Journal of Family Practice,* 1997; 44 (2): 138–144.

Van der Beek, EJ; van Dokkum, W; et al. "Thiamin, riboflavin, and vitamins $B_6$ and C: impact of combined restricted intake on functional performance in man."

*American Journal of Clinical Nutrition*, 1988; 48 (6): 1451–1462.

Zheng, JJ; Rosenberg, IH. "What is the nutritional status of the elderly?" *Geriatrics*, 1989; 44 (6): 57–58, 60, 63–64.

# · 2 ·

# The B Vitamins: One by One

As discussed in chapter 1, the B vitamins and their co-enzymes are closely related in terms of what functions they perform in the body and where in the diet they are found. Nevertheless, there exist some important—and fascinating—distinctions among them that deserve your attention. In this chapter, you'll discover all there is to know about the individual qualities of the B vitamins. Then, in chapter 3, we'll show you how to increase your daily intake of these important nutrients—and improve your health generally—by eating a balanced diet.

Before discussing the B vitamins in supplement form in this chapter, let's briefly explore some terms and concepts that will be helpful in this discussion.

# UNDERSTANDING VITAMIN SUPPLEMENTS

Because you're reading this book, chances are you're interested in learning more about, and taking advantage of, the power of vitamins to promote health and prevent disease. You're not alone. An estimated 100 million Americans spend about $6.5 billion a year on vitamin and mineral pills, up from $3 billion in 1990, according to the Council for Responsible Nutrition in Washington. This increase in use reflects both an increase in medical knowledge about the use of vitamins and minerals in the treatment and prevention of disease and a desire on the part of most Americans to seek more natural therapies for what ails them. Books like this one are designed to help people like you use vitamin and mineral supplements safely and effectively.

**The only term I hear consistently when it comes to vitamins is the Recommended Daily Allowance, or RDA. What is the RDA?**

Since 1943 or so, the Food and Nutrition Board of the National Research Council of the National Academy of Sciences have set forth standards called the Recommended Daily Allowances. Revised and updated on a regular basis, the RDAs represent the levels of nutrients necessary to meet or exceed the amount most people need of each of about twenty different vitamins, minerals, and proteins. For each nutrient, separate recommendations were made based on gender, age, and other factors.

The use of the RDA has been heavily criticized, since it does not take into account the needs of individuals in different health situations and the mounting evidence that vitamins and minerals play a critical role in the treatment and prevention of disease. Currently involved in a several-year study of the nutrient needs of men, women, and children, the board expects to release a comprehensive report, complete with updated nutritional guidelines, by the year 2001.

In the meantime, a piece of legislature called the Nutrition Labeling and Education Act of 1993 replaced the RDAs with the RDIs, also known as the Reference Daily Intakes. The RDIs are designed with the "average" man, woman, and child in mind—those who are healthy, able to absorb nutrients properly, exercise moderately, and are of average height and weight. As we've discussed, however, those who fall outside of such average categories usually require significantly more of one or more nutrients than the RDAs suggest. Furthermore, it is extremely difficult to obtain even these minimal requirements from the diet. That's why we—and most experts—encourage you to consider taking vitamin and mineral supplements in addition to eating a healthy, balanced diet.

### Does the government regulate vitamin safety?

In a broad sense, yes. The Federal Food and Drug Administration (FDA) is responsible for overseeing the safety and effectiveness of the ingredients in vitamin and mineral supplements and of the manufacturing process. The agency also monitors the way the manufacturers market and label supplements in order to protect consumers from false advertising claims about the nutrients' effects. However, the FDA does not put vitamin and mineral supplements under the same scrutiny—and expensive review process—as it does for substances designated as drugs or medications.

## What's the difference between organic, natural, and synthetic vitamins?

On a molecular level in the body, not much. All three types are equally effective. Organic vitamins are derived from animal and plant tissues and also from raw materials such as coal tar and wood pulp. Natural vitamins are organic but not all so-called "organic" vitamins are natural. Synthetic vitamins can be called organic as long as a molecule in the formula has at least one carbon atom. However, although vitamins labeled "natural" may contain substances created synthetically in a laboratory, they generally do not contain additives like coal tars, artificial coloring, preservatives, sugars, and starches, which are unnecessary and potentially harmful to the body. We recommend that you choose natural vitamins without additives.

## There are so many different vitamin potions out there. How do I start to supplement my diet?

A high-potency multivitamin that offers 100 percent or more of the RDIs for all or most essential nutrients is a great place to start. Multivitamin formulas combine a number of vitamins, minerals, and (often) amino acids in one tablet. Currently, a supplement is considered "high potency" if it contains 100 percent or more of the RDI for one or more nutrients.

Once you know you're consuming at least the minimum amounts of essential nutrients, you can look to see if you need to further increase your intake of a specific nutrient based on your personal health concerns, current dietary intake, and other factors. Based on the remarkable effects of the B vitamins, many people supplement their diets with a multivitamin plus a B-complex vitamin every day in order to reduce their chances of developing heart disease. In addition, women who suffer with premenstrual syndrome, for instance, may decide to take extra vitamin $B_6$ at certain times of their cycles to relieve uncomfortable symptoms.

**What about megadoses of vitamins? If a little bit is good, isn't a lot even better?**

Absolutely not. We do not recommend ever taking more than, say, two or three times the RDI for any nutrient without first consulting a doctor or qualified nutritionist. Although some claims can be made for the health benefits of taking very high doses of nutrients, most research proves that there is no significant benefit unless you're trying to address a very specific clinical deficiency. Bolstering your intake over the very limited values represented by the RDI, however, may very well help you avoid developing disease and treat some of the symptoms of marginal deficiencies you've already developed.

Second, we must emphasize that you should never take just one vitamin or mineral supplement without increasing—in relatively proportionate values—your intake of the others. Generally speaking, if you're taking no more than two or three times the RDI of any one nutrient, taking a good, high-potency multivitamin will make sure you don't create an imbalance by doing so.

**How soon can I expect to feel better after I start increasing my intake of B vitamins?**

Unlike many medications, vitamin therapy doesn't produce results overnight. In fact, it may take several weeks before the essential work vitamins perform produce noticeable effects. If, at the same time you start taking vitamins, you also start improving any other aspects of your health profile—exercising on a regular basis, reducing your stress levels, balancing your diet, eliminating toxins like cigarette smoke, caffeine, and food additives—the changes will occur that much more quickly.

**What is a good daily dose of B vitamins?**

How much of the B vitamins—and which of the B vitamins—you need depends on your own personal physiological makeup, your lifestyle, and your current health status. If you're a vigorous athlete, your body will need more of the nutrients that allow the muscles to do their powerful work. If you're pregnant, you'll want to increase your intake of a wide range of nutrients to feed your growing baby. We'll provide you with some general guidelines here and elsewhere, but if you have more questions, we suggest you talk to your doctor and/or a qualified nutritionist for extra help.

## UNDERSTANDING THE POWER OF THE Bs

In this section, we provide general descriptions of the eight B vitamins and their coenzymes. We tell you what functions each vitamin performs in the body, what a deficiency of each vitamin might produce and why such a deficiency might occur, and then list the current Recommended Daily Intakes.

When we refer to *therapeutic doses,* we mean those high doses doctors have used to treat severe deficiencies of the vitamin or to treat specific medical illnesses known to respond to high doses of the vitamin. As discussed, we recommend that you do not increase your intake of any B vitamin more than two or three times the RDI without first consulting a physician, and to always take a multivitamin at the same time in order to maintain a proper nutrient balance in your body.

Before we delve into the individual qualities of the various B vitamins, let's take a look at one of the easiest ways to obtain your minimum B vitamin requirements: the B-complex supplement.

## THE B-COMPLEX SUPPLEMENT

The vitamins in the B-complex supplement include $B_1$ (thiamin), $B_2$ (riboflavin), $B_3$ (niacin and niacinamide), pantothenic acid ($B_5$), $B_6$ (pyridoxine), $B_{12}$ (cobalamin), folic acid, and biotin. In addition, most B-complex supplements also include the B vitamin cofactors choline, inositol, and PABA. Although each B vitamin and cofactor has its own unique role to play in human physiology, they work together in such cooperation and are found together in nature so often that it makes sense to place them together in a supplement. We strongly suggest that you start on your journey to better health by taking either a multivitamin that contains 100 percent or more of the B vitamin RDIs or a B-complex supplement that provide the same. Once you've obtained the solid, nutritional base such supplements provide, you can further fine-tune your B vitamin requirements. We hope the information we provide below and throughout the book about the specific actions of each of the B vitamins will help you do just that.

## VITAMIN B₁

Perhaps better known as thiamin, vitamin $B_1$ acts as a co-enzyme participating in a variety of physiological activities. A severe deficiency causes a condition called beriberi, a disease that primarily affects the brain and nervous system, affecting mood and thought processes.

**Metabolic functions:** $B_1$, also known as thiamin, has several metabolic functions in the body. One of its primary functions is to convert carbohydrates into energy in the muscles and nerves. It is necessary for the formation of red blood cells and it is an important enzyme in the digestive process. Thiamin is also required for the production of acetylcholine, an important chemical called a neurotransmitter, which helps pass messages along one nerve cell to another.

**Potential causes of deficiency:** The modern American diet is a major culprit when it comes to the cause of thiamin deficiency. Because you need thiamin to metabolize carbohydrates, the more carbohydrates you eat, the more thiamin you use up. And that's true whether you eat a lot of junk food containing high levels of simple carbohydrates like sugar and white flour or eat a healthier diet of complex carbohydrates like whole wheat bread and pasta. Heavy coffee and tea drinkers also run a higher risk of having a thiamin deficiency since tannin, an ingredient in both substances, appears to interfere with thiamin absorption. Alcohol depletes thiamin, so much so that alcoholics suffer from a dementia called Wernicke-Korsakoff syndrome, which we discuss in depth in chapter 7.

Your diet may become depleted of thiamin because of your cooking methods: Thiamin is destroyed by the common food additive called sulfites and by moist heat such as that used to steam or boil vegetables. The use of alkalis such as baking soda with moist heat is especially damaging. Baking also is problematic: It can reduce the thiamin content of flour by 15 to 20 percent.

In addition, thiamin requirements rise whenever your body requires more energy than usual, such as during times of illness, stress, exercise, and pregnancy and lactation. Certain medications, particularly birth control pills, deplete thiamin as well.

**Deficiency symptoms:** Fatigue, forgetfulness, depression, headache, and confusion are among the first and most common symptoms of a thiamin deficiency, largely because of the vitamin's role in neurotransmission. Severe thiamin deficiency may result in anorexia, weight loss, gastrointestinal problems, cardiac abnormalities, and neurological disorders. Those at risk for thiamin deficiency include people with poor diets or with an inability to absorb nutrients properly, including the elderly, chronic alcohol abusers, and those with chronic gastrointestinal illnesses.

**Food sources:** Brewer's yeast, wheat germ, peanuts, sunflower seeds, pine nuts, organ meat, oatmeal, legumes such as lima beans and lentils, poultry, egg yolks, and fish are good sources of thiamin. In addition, many commercial grain products, such as bread and breakfast cereal, are fortified with thiamin.

**Reference Daily Intake:** The RDI for vitamin $B_1$ is 1.5 milligrams for men and women and 1.7 milligrams for pregnant and lactating women.

**Therapeutic dosages:** Therapeutic doses are considered to be between 50 and 200 milligrams per day. In cases of severe dementia traced to thiamin deficiency, doctors often prescribe up to 4 grams per day, but this is rare and not recommended without the supervision of a doctor trained in high-dose vitamin therapies (sometimes called *ortho-molecular medicine*).

**Toxicity levels and symptoms:** Thiamin has no known toxicity when taken orally in supplements or in the diet.

## I've heard thiamin deficiency and beriberi mentioned in connection to alcoholism. What's the connection?

In the United States today, the main population affected by thiamine deficiency severe enough to cause beriberi is that of chronic alcoholics. As discussed in chapter 1, alcoholics frequently suffer from malnutrition for two main reasons. First, they may simply not eat a proper diet due to lack of appetite. Second, alcohol can damage and irritate the stomach lining, thereby interfering with the ability of the digestive tract to absorb vitamins and minerals from ingested food. Finally, alcohol can interfere with the ability of the liver—which is also responsible for metabolizing alcohol—to metabolize certain nutrients, including thiamin, $B_6$, and folic acid.

In addition to classic beriberi, chronic alcohol abuse causes another $B_1$ deficiency syndrome called Wernicke-Korsakoff syndrome, which results in loss of short-term memory, disorientation, and gait disturbances. We'll discuss Wernicke-Korsakoff syndrome—and the therapeutic effects of increased vitamin B intake on this condition—further in chapter 7.

**I've heard about thiamin deficiency being responsible for constipation and other gastrointestinal disorders. Is that true?**

Like many of the other B vitamins, thiamin helps to efficiently metabolize the food you eat and is also responsible for maintaining proper muscle tone in the stomach. If you don't provide enough of this vitamin to your body, therefore, you may suffer symptoms of indigestion, constipation, and gastric distress.

## VITAMIN $B_2$ (RIBOFLAVIN): AN OVERVIEW

Vitamin $B_2$, better known as riboflavin, assists in a number of important chemical processes in the body.

**Metabolic functions:** The main function of riboflavin is to act as a precursor to two coenzymes essential to energy metabolism, helping cells to use oxygen to fuel their functions and processes. In fact, riboflavin is stored in the muscles and is used to fuel these tissues in times of physical exertion. In addition, riboflavin is involved in the metabolism of folic acid, niacin, and $B_6$. Riboflavin transforms amino acids into neurotransmitters, brain chemicals that allow memory, thought, and emotion to take place. Emerging research indicates that riboflavin may also act as an antioxidant, potentially helping to prevent cancer and control cholesterol buildup by helping to tame harmful free radicals.

**Potential causes of deficiency:** A deficiency in riboflavin alone is relatively rare, but it does occur. It often accompanies vitamin $B_1$ and niacin deficiencies. Severe and chronic alcohol abuse can lead to a deficiency, however, as can certain medications, including tranquilizers and antacids. Heavy coffee and tea drinkers are also at risk. In addition, it's important to realize that the vitamin is easily destroyed in the presence of light, so that foods stored in clear containers (glass milk bottles and clear jars that hold pasta and cereal) will lose vitamin $B_2$ quickly.

**Deficiency symptoms:** A riboflavin deficiency first affects the skin and other mucous membranes, causing soreness and burning of the lips, mouth, and tongue and burning and itching of the eyes, sensitivity to light, and loss of vision.

**Food sources:** The sources of the most concentrated amounts of riboflavin include milk products, organ meats (especially liver), and leafy green vegetables.

**Reference daily intake:** The Recommended Daily Allowances for men and women are about 1.5 milligrams; pregnant and lactating women should consume about 1.7 milligrams per day.

**Therapeutic dosages:** The therapeutic range for riboflavin is 50 to 200 milligrams per day but, again, you should discuss taking more than about three times the RDIs of any vitamin with your doctor before doing so.

**Toxicity levels and symptoms:** There are no toxicity levels for riboflavin; when intake exceeds 1.3 milligrams or so per day, greater quantities of the vitamin are excreted in the urine. However, in cases of increased need, such as illness or athletic training, less riboflavin is excreted. As is true for most of the other B vitamins, you can take about three times or more of the RDA of riboflavin without suffering any side effects or adverse consequences. At the same time, prolonged ingestion of large doses of just riboflavin can result in high losses of the other B vitamins, which is why it's so important to take a complete B-complex vitamin with any single B vitamin like riboflavin.

**I've heard about vitamin B$_2$ being used for the treatment of headaches. Is that true?**

As we'll discuss further in chapter 7, several studies link a B vitamin deficiency, and a riboflavin deficiency in particular, to the development of migraine headaches. For instance, on one double-blind study reported in *Neurology*, high doses (about 400 milligrams per day) of riboflavin significantly decreased the frequency of headaches in eighty migraine patients over a period of one year.

**What about arthritis? Is there a connection between riboflavin and that disease?**

Many experts believe that rheumatoid arthritis, a systemic disease that causes joint pain and disability, may be caused or exacerbated by the presence of free radicals. Since it appears that riboflavin has antioxidant properties, its use—along with other B vitamins and such antioxidant superstars as vitamins E, C, and beta-carotene—may help improve the condition.

## VITAMIN B$_3$ (NIACIN): AN OVERVIEW

One of the stars of the vitamin B world, vitamin B$_3$, commonly known as niacin, serves several metabolic functions and is used in therapeutic doses to treat a host of diseases, including, most effectively, high cholesterol and cardiovascular disease.

**Metabolic functions:** Vitamin $B_3$ comes in two forms: niacin and niacinamide, which have slightly different chemical makeups. Our bodies can make both forms from tryptophan, an amino acid found in protein. Both tryptophan and $B_3$ are important in the regulation of mood, and niacin has been used in a variety of psychiatric problems. Like many other B vitamins, niacin helps release energy from carbohydrates and aids in the breakdown of protein and fats. Its role in fat metabolism is so crucial that doctors prescribe it to reduce high levels of cholesterol and triglycerides. Vitamin $B_3$ also helps form certain hormones and is crucial to the production of red blood cells. Finally, vitamin $B_3$ also acts as a vasodilator, an agent that relaxes and widens the blood vessels, which makes it helpful in the treatment of other cardiovascular problems.

**Potential causes of deficiency:** Severe niacin deficiencies are rare, but they do occur in alcoholics or others who are malnourished. Because vitamin $B_6$ is needed to convert tryptophan into niacin in the body, a deficiency of that vitamin can result in a niacin deficiency.

**Deficiency symptoms:** Early signs of vitamin $B_3$ deficiencies are largely mental and emotional, including depression, loss of memory, and feelings of apprehension. As the condition worsens, hysteria and confusion can ensue. In addition, skin rashes and gastrointestinal disorders may develop. Finally, classic severe niacin deficiency disease—also known as pellagra—is characterized by the "four Ds": dermatitis, diarrhea, dementia, and then death.

**Food sources:** You can find plentiful stores of vitamin $B_3$ in animal protein products, including beef, pork, fish, milk, eggs, and cheese. Whole wheat, potatoes, tomatoes, and carrots also contain $B_3$.

**Reference daily intake:** In order to stave off overt $B_3$ deficiency, you need to consume about 20 milligrams of $B_3$ every day.

**Therapeutic dosages:** Therapeutic doses range from 50 to 200 milligrams a day or more.

**Toxicity levels and symptoms:** Daily doses of up to about 1,000 milligrams appear to be safe, but niacin is likely to be toxic for some people who consume several grams of the vitamin. Too much niacin may cause depression in some people, and other toxic symptoms include nausea, diarrhea, and irregular heartbeat. For those who suffer from gout, too much niacin can increase their risks of suffering an attack. Large doses may also cause liver damage because the liver metabolizes vitamin $B_3$, and a doctor should monitor intake of any dose much higher than two or three times the RDI. Niacinamide seems to have less of these toxic effects than the niacin form.

**You say here that there are few side effects from niacin. But my father used to suffer from niacin flushes when he took it. Isn't that dangerous?**

What you're describing is a fairly common—but usually quite harmless—reaction to the vasodilative action of niacin. This action not only causes blood to rush to the face, but also triggers the release of histamine, a body chemical involved in the allergic response. Histamine can cause itchiness as well as flushing. Usually the reaction lasts for just about fifteen minutes or so and, although quite uncomfortable, is not dangerous. Certain synthetic forms of niacin, particularly a form called inositol hexaniacinate, have the positive effects of niacin without the flushing. Niacinamide also does not cause flushing, but it is not as useful as niacin in lowering cholesterol and dilating blood vessels.

## Are there any people who shouldn't take niacin supplements?

Anyone suffering with peptic ulcers, liver disease, gout, or significant heart rhythm disturbances should take supplementary niacin only with the advice of a physician.

## I've never heard of pellagra. Was it ever a common condition?

Prior to the 1940s, a deficiency in vitamin $B_3$ frequently resulted in a disease called pellagra, which causes diarrhea, skin disorders, fatigue, muscular weakness, and mental disorders. At the turn of the century in the American South, this ailment afflicted more than 100,000 people, largely because their diets consisted mainly of cornmeal. Today, thanks largely to the presence of foods fortified with $B_3$, the disease is almost nonexistent in the industrialized world, even in poor areas.

## I've heard about niacin in relation to heart disease. What's the connection?

In chapter 5, we discuss the various ways that niacin can be used to treat cardiovascular disease. In large doses, for instance, niacin lowers serum cholesterol concentrations and doctors now prescribe a time-release formula of niacin to treat the disease. Another cardiovascular disease niacin may help alleviate is Raynaud's disease, a painful condition that results from the abnormal constriction of blood vessels in very hot or, more commonly, very cold conditions. Not only does this cause tingling and aching, but it can also lead to localized infections in the fingernails and toenails that can be quite nasty.

**Are there other conditions doctors use niacin to treat?**

Studies on niacin indicate that it may suppress the development of type I diabetes. Other findings suggest that it may also play a role in autoimmune diseases such as rheumatoid arthritis and chronic ulcerative colitis. Niacin supplements may also reduce the incidence of asthma-induced wheezing, perhaps because this nutrient prevents the release of histamine, a biochemical normally released during allergic reactions. Harvard University researchers found that people who got the most niacin in their diets were significantly less likely to have bronchitis or wheezing than people who got the least. Lower blood levels of niacin were also linked to wheezing.

A few decades ago, Dr. Stanley Kaufmann chronicled the use of niacinamide to treat osteoarthritis, particularly in the knees. This treatment is still prescribed by some nutritionally oriented physicians.

Finally, some research indicates that vitamin $B_3$ can help improve some types of schizophrenia. In chapter 7, we'll explore this issue in more depth, but for now it might interest you to know that some doctors use high doses of niacin and niacinamide to treat serious mental and neurological diseases.

## PANTOTHENIC ACID (VITAMIN B₅)

Pantothenic acid occurs in all living cells and is present in all yeast, molds, and bacteria. The body can produce its own pantothenic acid. Or, more correctly, the bacterial flora that live in our intestines produce vitamin $B_5$ that is then absorbed into the body.

**Metabolic functions:** Like its other B cohorts, pantothenic acid acts as a coenzyme in carbohydrate, protein, and fat and cholesterol metabolism. In fact, before any sugar can be burned for fuel, it must be converted to a substance called acetyl coenzyme A, and you must have enough pantothenic acid for that conversion to occur. It also aids in the synthesis of hormones and in the production of hemoglobin, the oxygen-carrying pigment in red blood cells, and it helps produce two neurotransmitters, sphingosine and acetylcholine, which make it crucial for the function of thought processes and the regulation of mood.

Pantothenic acid is concentrated in the adrenal glands of the body, where it plays a critical role in the body's proper response to stress.

**Potential causes of deficiency:** Because pantothenic acid is found in many different foods, overt deficiencies are rare, especially now that many grain products are fortified with B vitamins. However, trying to get all you need from the food you eat may be difficult unless you concentrate on getting enough of these fortified products. More than 33 percent of the pantothenic acid content of meat is lost during cooking, and 50 percent is lost by the milling of flour (which is one reason that the fortification process is necessary). In times of stress or illness, or if you drink copious amounts of alcohol, coffee, or tea, you may require more pantothenic acid along with other B vitamins.

**Deficiency symptoms:** A deficiency of this vitamin alone is unlikely unless severe B-complex vitamin malnutrition exists. Symptoms include the sensations of tingling in the hands and feet, loss of appetite, depression, fatigue, insomnia, vomiting, and muscular cramping or weakness. Severe deficiency symptoms include vomiting, severe abdominal cramps, and physical and mental depression.

**Food sources:** Chicken, fish, beef, pork, organ meat, brewer's yeast, oatmeal, and hazelnuts are especially good sources of pantothenic acid. Avocados, cauliflower, and leafy green vegetables such as kale and spinach also contain significant quantities of pantothenic acid.

**Reference daily intake:** No RDI has yet been set for pantothenic acid, but from 4 to 7 milligrams per day is generally considered adequate.

**Therapeutic dosages:** The common therapeutic range is between 50 and 250 milligrams per day, but doses of up to 1,000 milligrams per day have been used without incident.

**Toxicity levels and symptoms:** So far, no toxic effects have been noted with the use of pantothenic acid. However, people with rheumatoid arthritis should consult their physician before taking larger doses.

**What other health conditions can pantothenic acid help treat or prevent?**

Pantothenic acid, along with another vitamin B coenzyme called CoQ10, appears to help prevent the accumulation of fatty acids within the heart muscle, thereby reducing the risk of heart disease. We'll discuss this in more depth in chapter 5. Some research indicates that pantothenic acid is vital to the healthy functioning of the immune system. In his book, *All About B Vitamins*, Burt Berkson, M.D., Ph.D., a practitioner of integrative medicine and president of the Integrative Medical Centers of New Mexico, reports that people who take high doses of pantothenic acid suffer from fewer herpes virus, Epstein-Barr virus, and shingles infections. It appears that pantothenic acid is essential to the health of the thymus and antibody production.

Probably because of its positive effects on the stress response, pantothenic acid is useful in the treatment of allergies. Nutritional prescriptions frequently include higher doses of vitamin $B_5$ during allergy season, along with smaller doses of the other B vitamins and of the mineral zinc.

**Who shouldn't take extra $B_5$?**

Anyone taking any medication—over-the-counter or prescription—should not take pantothenic acid without consulting his or her doctor. And there is a special warning to those who have Parkinson's disease. If you're taking pure levodopa, do not take pantothenic acid; even small amounts will nullify levodopa's effects. However, if you're taking the more common combination of carbidopa-levodopa, pantothenic acid will not interfere with its metabolism or use.

**I've heard that some people take pantothenic acid in the winter. Why is that?**

As you may remember, pantothenic acid is required for the conversion of a substance called coenzyme A into energy and heat. You have a greater need for more of this energy, and thus more pantothenic acid, in colder weather.

## VITAMIN B$_6$: AN OVERVIEW

Also known as pyroxidine, vitamin B$_6$ is perhaps best known as a treatment for premenstrual syndrome, but recent research indicates that it has as many functions in the body as its other vitamin B brethren. In fact, this nutrient is involved in roughly 100 enzymatic reactions.

**Metabolic functions:** B$_6$ is a cofactor for many enzymes involved in the breakdown of fat, protein, and carbohydrates in the body. The release of glycogen for energy from the muscles and liver requires B$_6$. In addition, B$_6$ aids in the conversion of the amino acid tryptophan to the neurotransmitter serotonin, an important neurotransmitter involved in the regulation of sleep and mood. It's also essential for the synthesis and proper action of RNA and DNA and is necessary for the metabolism of amino acids, which are the building blocks of protein. It plays a special role in keeping homocysteine levels at a healthy level. Vitamin B$_6$ plays a role in the production of all cells and must be present for the production of red blood cells and cells of the immune system. B$_6$ has been successful in treating a range of conditions, including premenstrual syndrome, carpal tunnel syndrome, insomnia, irritability, and depression.

**Potential causes of deficiency:** As is true for the other B vitamins, severe $B_6$ deficiency may occur in certain high-risk populations, especially the malnourished elderly, chronic alcoholics, and those with cancer or other chronic illnesses that require medication with certain toxic drugs. Marginal deficiencies may occur in anyone who doesn't eat a healthy, balanced diet consisting of plentiful fresh fruits and vegetables, whole grains, and lean protein. Drugs like oral contraceptives and seizure medications also deplete the body's $B_6$.

**Deficiency symptoms:** In the early stages of $B_6$ deficiency, symptoms include hair loss, cracks around the mouth and eyes, dermatitis, numbness and tingling in the arms and legs, and difficulty with concentration. As the deficiency progresses, arthritis, heart disorders, and anemia may ensue. Because $B_6$ is important in the regulation of the toxic chemical homocysteine, a long-standing deficiency may contribute to cardiovascular diseases such as arteriosclerosis, heart attack, and stroke.

Dr. John Ellis studied the relationship of vitamin $B_6$ deficiency to a complex of high cholesterol, swelling of the hands and feet (particularly during pregnancy or premenstrually), and tingling of the extremities. He treated these people with higher doses of pyridoxine.

Most of the reactions involving vitamin $B_6$ also involve the use of the mineral magnesium, and it is recommended to take magnesium whenever $B_6$ is being given. Sometimes, if symptoms don't respond to vitamin $B_6$, they will respond to added magnesium.

**Food sources:** The best sources of vitamin $B_6$ include meat, organ meat, chicken, and fish. Bananas, walnuts, navy beans, sunflower seeds, and wheat germ are also excellent sources.

**Reference daily intake:** The current RDI for $B_6$ is about 2.0 milligrams/day for men and 1.6 milligrams for women, and 2.2 milligrams for pregnant and lactating women. However, $B_6$ requirements are dependent on protein metabolism, so the more protein you consume, the more $B_6$ you need.

**Therapeutic dosages:** Therapeutic doses of $B_6$ range from 30 to 500 milligrams/day.

**Toxicity levels and symptoms:** Doses of more than 250 milligrams/day may cause nerve damage, so should only be taken under a doctor's care.

**My daughter swears that vitamin $B_6$ helps her sleep better. Why would that be true?**

Vitamin $B_6$ may promote better sleep because of its role in the production of neurotransmitters, primarily serotonin. In turn, the presence of serotonin in sufficient quantities triggers the release of melatonin, a hormone known for its sleep-enhancing effects.

## VITAMIN $B_{12}$: AN OVERVIEW

Vitamin $B_{12}$, also known as cobalamin, is unique in the vitamin world because it also contains an essential mineral: cobalt. It also cannot be made synthetically but must be grown, like penicillin, from bacteria and molds.

**Metabolic functions:** Stored in the liver, vitamin $B_{12}$ is essential for proper nerve function, blood cell formation, memory, and the metabolism of fat, carbohydrate, and protein. It also helps iron function better in the body and helps the body better absorb and use vitamin A. As is true for folic acid, it is especially important in the formation of DNA and RNA, the body's genetic material. Finally, along with vitamin $B_6$ and folic acid, vitamin $B_{12}$ aids in the safe conversion of homocysteine into other, nontoxic substances.

**Potential causes of deficiency:** Although a poor diet and medications can interfere with your ability to obtain sufficient vitamin $B_{12}$, most deficiencies result from the inability to absorb enough of the vitamin once ingested because of a lack of an intrinsic factor, an essential gastric secretion. Up to 10 percent of the elderly have deficiencies of vitamin $B_{12}$ accompanied by neuropsychiatric disorders such as depression, Alzheimer's disease and other dementias, and anxiety.

Natural-oriented physicians treated childhood asthma and allergic problems with vitamin $B_{12}$ shots until the 1950s. It was felt that these conditions related to a lowered hydrochloric acid, which led to a lower $B_{12}$. This strategy is still used by nutritionally based physicians today, as it has never been disproven.

**Deficiency symptoms:** Symptoms of mild $B_{12}$ deficiencies include fatigue and difficulty in concentration.

**Food sources:** Vitamin $B_{12}$ is a product of bacterial metabolism. The best food sources of vitamin $B_{12}$ are animal products such as beef, chicken, organ meat, fish, and eggs. Plants do not contain active forms of $B_{12}$, which makes it almost impossible for vegetarians to obtain all the $B_{12}$ they need from their diet alone. People on strict vegetarian diets usually include foods that use bacterial fermentation, such as tempeh, or they supplement $B_{12}$ in an oral form.

**Reference daily intake:** The RDI for vitamin $B_{12}$ is 3.0 micrograms per day.

**Therapeutic dosages:** Doses of up to 5,000 micrograms/day are not uncommon for therapeutic purposes.

**Toxicity levels and symptoms:** Vitamin $B_{12}$ is extremely safe, and no toxicity from even very high doses of the nutrient has been reported.

### What is pernicious anemia?

An extreme deficiency of $B_{12}$ can result in pernicious anemia, a condition characterized by production of red blood cells that have impaired oxygen-carrying capacities. Pernicious anemia can cause fatigue, gastrointestinal disturbances, partial loss of coordination of the fingers, feet, and limbs, loss of appetite, and in severe cases, death. Poor intake and absorption of $B_{12}$ can also lead to neurological problems, especially among the elderly. Very low blood $B_{12}$ levels can result in other neurological disorders, including depression and tingling of the extremities.

## FOLIC ACID

Folic acid, also known as folate or folacin, is best known for its ability to help prevent neural tube birth defects. It also helps to fight cancer and reduce risk of heart disease.

**Metabolic functions:** The body requires folic acid in order to properly form red blood cells and metabolize protein. It also allows cells to grow and divide and works within the brain to promote good emotional health. It also stimulates the production of HCl, which helps protect against intestinal parasites and food poisoning. Synthesis of cysteine—and not the toxic homocysteine—from methionine is also dependent on folic acid, which makes it an essential nutrient in the fight against cardiovascular disease, Alzheimer's disease, osteoporosis, and other conditions affected by high homocysteine levels.

**Potential causes of deficiency:** Poor dietary intake of folic acid–rich food is the primary reason for a folic acid deficiency. Certain medications, including birth control pills, antacids, and antibiotics also deplete the body of folic acid. Heat will destroy folic acid, so cooking will rob food of this important nutrient.

**Deficiency symptoms:** Long-term deficiency of folic acid can result in fatigue, gastrointestinal disturbances (especially diarrhea), impaired nutrient absorption, metabolic disturbances, mouth sores and other mucous membrane irritations, and pernicious anemia. Cervical cell changes (cervical dysplasia) are also more common in women who are deficient in folic acid. Because of its role in the formation of DNA, all women of childbearing age are urged to maintain sufficient levels of folic acid in order to prevent birth defects in their children should they become pregnant.

**Food sources:** Citrus fruits and juices, leafy dark green vegetables, wheat germ, and legumes are good sources of folic acid.

**Reference daily intake:** The RDI for folic acid is 400 micrograms/day.

**Therapeutic dosages:** Doses ranging from 400 micrograms to 10 milligrams/day have been used clinically, but a more common therapeutic range is 400 to 1,000 micrograms/day.

**Toxicity levels and symptoms:** Because folic acid supplementation may mask the symptoms of $B_{12}$ deficiency, most experts don't recommend that you take more than 400 micrograms of the vitamin per day. However, as long as you make sure to take a B-complex vitamin containing $B_{12}$, such a problem shouldn't exist. Very high doses—more than 15 grams per day—can cause insomnia, irritability, and gastrointestinal problems.

### Is there a connection between folic acid and cancer?

There appears to be. The occurrence of precancerous colon polyps is associated with low folic acid levels. Similarly, it may play a role in the prevention of oral, uterine, and cervical cancers as well. We'll discuss this connection further in chapter 6.

## BIOTIN (VITAMIN $B_7$)

Also known as vitamin H, biotin is produced in the intestines by bacteria as well as being found in the diet. It is an essential nutrient that appears in trace amounts in all animal and plant tissue.

**Metabolic functions:** Biotin helps to form fatty acids, which are important in the production of keratin, the protein that forms healthy skin, hair, and nails. It also works with the other B vitamins in metabolizing proteins, fat, and carbohydrates.

**Potential causes of deficiency:** Use of antibiotics destroys the friendly bacteria in the intestines that produce biotin, which can lead to a deficiency. In addition, people who eat large amounts of raw egg whites are also at risk. Egg whites contain a substance called avidin, which binds to biotin in the intestine and prevents its absorption.

**Deficiency symptoms:** Brittle nails, hair loss, and skin disorders—particularly dermatitis and eczema—may be among the first symptoms of a biotin deficiency, but the substance is essential to so many different body systems that there may be others, including depression, nausea, muscle pains, anemia, and high cholesterol.

**Food sources:** Some rich sources of biotin include brewer's yeast, pork and lamb liver, whole grains, egg yolks, sardines, soybeans, lentils, and cauliflower.

**Reference daily intake:** No RDI has been set for biotin, but a range of 30 to 100 micrograms/day is suggested.

**Therapeutic dosages:** You can take up to 300 to 600 micrograms/day to treat a known deficiency or an ailment that responds to treatment with biotin.

**Toxicity levels and symptoms:** No toxicity symptoms have been reported with biotin, primarily because—like most other water-soluble vitamins—any excess is excreted in the urine.

**I've read about biotin and diabetes. Is there a connection?**

For reasons not yet understood, people with type II diabetes (non–insulin dependent) tend to have significantly lower biotin levels than people without the disease. When Japanese researchers studied the biotin and blood sugar levels of people with diabetes, they found that the higher someone's blood sugar, the lower his level of biotin. They also noted that people with diabetes have significantly lower biotin levels than people who don't have the disease. Researchers then gave 9 milligrams (9,000 micrograms) of biotin to eighteen people with diabetes every day for a month and found that their glucose levels fell to nearly half their original levels.

## VITAMIN B COFACTORS

Although not exactly vitamins, the following substances work with the B vitamins to perform their metabolic actions within the body. Generally speaking, as long as you consume a multivitamin or B-complex supplement, you'll obtain adequate levels of these cofactors.

### CHOLINE

Like its B vitamin counterparts, choline plays an important role in the metabolism of proteins, carbohydrates, and, more particularly, of fat. In addition, it helps produce acetylcholine, a neurotransmitter that permits nerve cells to transmit messages to and from the brain. These functions make it essential to the proper development and function of the brain and central nervous system, and a deficit of this nutrient may be implicated in the development of Alzheimer's disease and other neurological disorders.

## INOSITOL

Inositol is found in tissues of the brain and nervous system, bones, reproductive organs, and the heart as well as in cell membranes. It appears to play an important role in nerve transmission, the regulation of certain enzymes, and in the manufacture and transport of fats.

## PARA-AMINOBENZOIC ACID (PABA)

You probably know this vitamin B relative best as an ingredient of sunscreen that helps shield your skin from the potential damage of ultraviolet radiation. Doctors also use it to treat vitiligo, a condition characterized by discoloration or depigmentation of some areas of the skin, and to treat burns and other wounds. Internally, PABA also has important functions, such as stimulating intestinal bacteria, enabling them to produce folic acid, which in turn aids in the production of pantothenic acid. As a coenzyme, it helps the body break down and use proteins as well as helps to produce red blood cells.

### How much of these substances do I need every day?

The Food and Nutrition Board has not set standard RDIs for these substances. Generally speaking, you can derive all you need of each of these cofactors by taking a vitamin B-complex supplement and by eating a diet rich in B vitamins like the one we'll describe in the next chapter.

## REFERENCES FOR CHAPTER TWO

Allen, R; Stabler, S; Savage, D; et al. "Metabolic abnormalities in cobalamin (vitamin $B_{12}$) and folate deficiency." *FASEB J* 1993; 1344–1353.

Bendich, A. "Vitamin supplement safety issues." *Nutrition Report*, 1993; 11: 57–64.

Bower, C; Stanley, F; Nicol, D. "Maternal folate status and risk for neural tube defects. *Annals of the New York Academy of Sciences*, 1993; 678: 146–155.

Brantigan, CO. "Folate supplementation and the risk of masking vitamin $B_{12}$ deficiency." *Journal of the American Medical Association*, 1997; 277: 884.

Butterworth, CE: Tamura, T. "Folic acid safety and toxicity: a brief review." *American Journal of Clinical Nutrition*, 1989; 50: 353–358.

Campbell, NR. "How safe are folic acid supplements?" *Archives of Internal Medicine*, 1996; 156: 1638–1644.

Eastman, C; Gullarte, T. "Vitamin $B_6$, kynurenines, and central nervous system function." *Journal of Nutritional Biochemistry*, 1992; 3: 618–631.

Freedman, M; Tighe, S; Damato, D; et al. "Vitamin $B_{12}$ in Alzheimer's disease. *Canadian Journal of Neurology*, 1986; 13: 183.

Guilarte, T. "Vitamin $B_6$ and cognitive development: recent research findings from human and animal studies." *Nutrition Review*, 1993; 51: 193–198.

Meador, K; Nichols, M; Franke, P; et al. "Evidence for a central cholinergic effect on high-dose thiamin." *Annals of Neurology*, 1993; 34: 724–726.

Mock, D; Johnson, S; Holman, R. "Effects of biotin deficiency on serum fatty acid composition." *Journal of Nutrition*, 1988; 118: 342–348.

O'Keeffe, S; Tormey, W; et al. "Thiamin deficiency in hospitalized elderly patients." *Gerontology*, 1994; 40: 18–24.

Prasad, A; et al. "Effect of oral contraceptive agents on nutrients. II: Vitamins." *American Journal of Clinical Nutrition*, 1975; 28: 385.

Sauberlich, H. "Interactions: vitamins, minerals and hazardous elements." *Annals of the New York Academy of Sciences*, 1980; 355: 80–97.

Schoenen, J, et al. "Effectiveness of high-dose riboflavin in migraine prophylaxis. A randomized controlled trial." *Neurology*, 1995; 50: 996–1002.

Vermaak, W; Ubbink, J; Barnard, H. "Vitamin $B_6$ nutrition status and cigarette smoking." *American Journal of Clinical Nutrition*, 1990; 51: 1058–1061.

# · 3 ·

# Your Diet: Maximizing Your B Vitamin Intake

Providing your body with at least the minimum requirements of the B vitamins with your diet your alone is not
impossible if you eat a healthy, balanced diet. Easier said
than done, right? In fact, if you have trouble understanding
and then meeting the goal of eating a healthy diet, you're
not alone. Millions of Americans are overweight and—
ironically—undernourished because they're eating the
wrong kinds of food in the wrong amounts.

In this chapter, we'll outline for you the standard healthy
diet that—if you follow it—offers you the best chance of
meeting your basic nutritional needs. We'll then explore in
more depth the foods that are especially rich in the B vitamins. As you know by now, these vitamins are vital to
the health of your cardiovascular system, your brain and
nervous system, your chances (if you're a woman of childbearing age) of having a healthy baby, and to a host of
other body systems and processes.

## THE BASICS

To revisit the analogy of the human body as laboratory brought up in chapter 1, you can think of the food you eat as the chemicals your laboratory needs to cook up health and vitality. It requires about forty different essential nutrients to accomplish that. These nutrients include oxygen, water, protein, carbohydrates, fats, and a host of vitamins and minerals. Your body receives oxygen from the air you breathe, and without it you could not survive for more than a few minutes. Although most of us take oxygen for granted, study after study proves that the more oxygen you supply to your body's cells, by breathing deeply and circulating more oxygen-rich blood during aerobic exercise, the better.

Water, which is found in almost everything we eat and drink, is another substance most of us take for granted. Water regulates body temperature, circulation, and excretion, and aids in digestion. It bathes virtually all of our cells in moisture, and it is especially vital to the health and beauty of skin tissue. Nevertheless, few of us drink the sixty-four ounces of water our body needs every day to stay healthy.

The other thirty-eight or so essential nutrients are found in the foods we eat. What we call a balanced diet is one that contains the appropriate amount—not too little and not too much—of those nutrients on a daily basis. In addition, a balanced diet also involves providing the right amount of calories—the energy value of food—to maintain proper body weight. A calorie represents the amount of energy the body needs to burn in order to use up that bit of food; any excess energy is stored as fat.

Now, how can you make sure that you get as many of those thirty-eight essential nutrients in your diet every day?

Well, In 1989, the United States Department of Agriculture and the U.S. Department of Health and Human Services released dietary recommendations in the form of the Food Guide Pyramid, a visual and practical guide to a healthy, balanced diet. However, this plan emphasizes eating high levels of carbohydrates, which may cause weight gain and insulin resistance in some people. Other versions of the plan, including the Mediterranean Food Pyramid, concentrate on including more olive oil, lean protein, and lots of fruits and vegetables. While we encourage you to investigate the fundamentals of a healthy diet on your own, the Food Pyramid will get you started.

## THE BASICS OF NUTRITION

Most of us grew up with the idea that a balanced diet included equal amounts of four food groups: dairy, grains, meats, and fruits and vegetables. Today, we know that eating right involves a few more categories and a little more finesse.

First of all, food is nourishment. The nutrients in the food you eat are the catalysts for millions of major and minor miracles—the beating of your heart, the birth of an idea, the appreciation of smell and taste, the movement of the blood through the vessels—that take place within the body. But second—and this is an important point—food is also a source of pleasure. We do not eat merely to ingest the various vitamins, minerals, and other substances we need to survive. Instead, eating is a supremely sensual activity: We smell food's aromas, taste its flavors, admire its colors and textures, and feel its consistency in our mouths. Depending on the circumstances, our sense of hearing is also stimulated by the conversation of our tablemates or the sounds of dinner music.

In this book, however, we're concentrating on giving your body the raw materials it needs to survive and thrive. One way to look at the diet is through the Food Guide Pyramid, a plan put forth by the U.S. Department of Agriculture. The plan organizes the food you'll eat into six different categories and shows us how much—proportionately speaking—of each type of food we should eat every day. (Again, there are several versions of this plan, including the Mediterranean diet that emphasizes—even more than this plan—the importance of lean protein, fresh vegetables and fruits, and monounsaturated fats like olive oil. However, the standard Food Guide Pyramid should get you started on creating a more healthful diet.) Let's take a look:

• *Complex carbohydrates* (6 to 11 servings a day). According to the Food Guide Pyramid, complex carbohydrates should make up the bulk of your daily caloric intake. Carbohydrates are substances that provide the body with energy and fiber. Whole-grain bread, pasta, and rice are the primary forms of complex carbohydrates. However, once again, we want to emphasize that too many bread products, particularly white rice, pasta, and bread, may actually cause you to gain weight and perhaps put you at risk for the development of insulin resistance or diabetes. We suggest that you keep in mind that the complex carbohydrates group also consists of vegetables and fruits, which are far better to emphasize than white-flour products.

• *Protein* (2 to 4 servings a day). Protein is the major component of our muscles, bones, teeth, and certain cell components. The average adult needs to consume about 55 grams of protein per day, or about the amount supplied in about 4 ounces of lean meat, chicken, or fish. Among the most healthful sources of protein are cold-water fish such as mackerel, herring, and salmon and, as far as the B vitamins go, organ meats like liver and kidneys. Several vegetable sources of protein, including some beans and legumes, provide other nutrients in addition to protein that make them good choices as well.

• *Fruit* (2 to 4 servings per day). The luscious sweetness of a peach, the richness of a banana, the tartness of fresh cherries . . . In addition to the pleasure we get from the flavor and texture of fruit, our bodies receive some essential nutrients from this food, including antioxidants and flavonoids, two substances that work to keep body cells healthy.

• *Vegetables* (3 to 5 servings, or more, per day). Vegetables provide the body with a wide variety of vitamins and minerals essential for its proper functioning, as well as fiber to keep the digestive tract in good working order.

• *Dairy products* (2 to 3 servings per day). Low-fat or skim milk, cheese, and yogurt are important to include in our daily diets because they contain calcium, magnesium, and vitamin D—all essential for the building and maintenance of our bones and muscles. For those of us who have difficulty digesting dairy products, there are other equally nutritious sources of these nutrients. Leafy green vegetables contain lots of calcium and magnesium, for instance, while fish and the rays of the sun provide us with vitamin D. As you'll see in the next section, milk and milk products also provide a fair amount of some of the B vitamins.

• *Fats and sugars* (sparingly). From the foods listed above, we receive all the fat and sugar we need to live. However, as most of us can attest, fat and sugar, especially in combination, taste good. As long as you limit the amount of these substances you eat on a regular basis, you should feel free to enjoy an occasional feast.

If you follow this rough outline—cutting way back on fat and sugar, eating more fresh fruits and vegetables, lean protein, and complex carbohydrates—it's likely you'll obtain at least the minimum daily requirements for your nutrients.

**I understand the concept of the Food Guide Pyramid, but the one thing it doesn't tell you is what "one serving" is. I think I eat the right proportion of carbohydrates to fat, but I still seem to gain weight. Can you help?**

Sure—and don't feel silly for asking, because portion control is perhaps the biggest problem Americans have when it comes to weight control. Here's a rundown of what one serving of each type of food really is:

*Bread, Cereal, Rice, and Pasta*

• 1 slice of bread

• 1 ounce of cereal

• ½ cup of cooked rice or pasta

*Vegetables*

• 1 cup of raw leafy vegetables

• ½ cup of other vegetables, cooked or chopped raw

• ¾ cup of vegetable juice

*Fruit*

- 1 medium apple, banana, or orange

- ½ cup of chopped or canned fruit

- ¾ cup of fruit juice

*Milk, Yogurt, and Cheese*

- 1 cup of milk or yogurt

- 1½ ounces of natural cheese

- 2 ounces of processed cheese

*Meat, Poultry, Fish, Dry Beans, Eggs, and Nuts*

- 2 to 3 ounces of cooked lean meat, poultry, or fish

- ½ cup of cooked dry beans

- 1 egg

- 2 tablespoons of peanut butter

As you can see, it's all too easy to overeat, and even if you're eating the right kinds of food, that can mean weight gain. The average serving of pasta, for instance, is about 2 cups or four times what one serving truly represents. Instead of consuming about 200 calories per serving, you'd be downing a total of 800 calories—and that's not counting the butter, sauce, meat, or cheese with which you top your pasta.

**Do you have other tips to help me work this pyramid plan to my best advantage?**

Sure thing. Here are some tips that might help you get the most out of your diet:

• *Try to eat five to six small meals a day.* The more often you eat, the less hungry you'll be and the less food you'll eat at each meal. That means you'll be better able to digest your food, and you'll absorb the nutrients you provide the body more efficiently. Try to eat breakfast, a midmorning snack, lunch, an afternoon snack, dinner, and a before-bedtime snack—all consisting of low-fat, low-sugar, high-nutrient foods, of course!

• *Halve your intake of oils and fats while doubling your intake of fresh vegetables and whole grains.* Unfortunately, most Americans eat too much of the wrong kinds of fats, namely processed vegetable oils, which provide calories but no other nutrients. However, monounsaturated fat such as that found in olive oil can be beneficial to your health if used in moderation. Instead of applying a fat-laden dollop of salad dressing on your greens, dribble a little garlic-flavored olive oil and a squirt of lemon. You'll still get that great smooth feeling that fat brings to food, but you'll actually be doing your heart and vessels some good.

• *Consume all good things in moderation.* Unless you have specific food allergies or other medical problems, no food should be off limits to you. Instead of spending precious time, energy, and stress avoiding foods that society considers bad, you should work on integrating small amounts of those forbidden foods into your diet.

• *Plan and cook ahead.* If you make an effort to organize your eating by creating a menu for the week, shopping, and even cooking ahead of time, it's likely that you'll enjoy your mealtimes more and broaden the variety of foods you eat. You'll thus also increase your chances of getting your basic RDIs—including those for the B vitamins—from your diet.

• *Add variety to your diet.* By eating lots of different kinds of foods during the day, you'll not only improve your chances of meeting your RDIs, you're also likely to find yourself enjoying your diet more than ever. At least once a week, try a new food—an exotic fruit or vegetable, for instance—or cook a different dish.

• *Eat foods that leave you feeling healthy and well.* Pay attention to how you feel after you eat your meals. If you're often groggy and uncomfortable, you may be eating too much, failing to eat a balanced diet, or consuming food that doesn't agree with your particular body makeup. Nutritious food, prepared well and eaten in a relaxed atmosphere, should nourish you, body and soul.

## What about exercise? How important is that to my general health?

Ah, exercise. Good question. Without exercise, your body simply will not be healthy or vital—or at least it won't be for long. Although exercise is often perceived as a painful, tedious process, especially by those who need it most, properly performed, regular exercise soon becomes a positive, life-enhancing habit. It allows you to connect with your body in an intimate way, as you feel your muscles grow stronger, your heart beat harder, and the tension of the day slip away.

Although it goes far beyond the scope of this book to

give you a comprehensive overview of the importance of physical activity, here's a brief look at the three basic components of an overall fitness program, each one as important as the other:

- *Cardiovascular fitness.* Also known as aerobic exercise, cardiovascular exercise uses large muscle groups to get the heart pumping and the lungs filling with oxygen. With aerobic exercise, your body learns to burn fat more efficiently as fuel. Among the best aerobic exercises are walking, jogging, aerobic dance, stair-climbing, and step classes.

- *Strength training.* Also known as anaerobic exercise, strength training is just as important to overall fitness as aerobic exercise. Muscle is more metabolically active than fat, which simply means that the body must burn more calories to feed and nourish muscle tissues than it does to maintain fat.

- *Flexibility and balance.* Most Americans, even those who consider themselves to be in top physical condition, neglect flexibility. Part of the reason may lie in the non-competitive nature of stretching—there are no times to beat or weight limits to surpass. However, practicing yoga or learning other ways to stretch and lengthen your muscles is one of the best ways to attain a state of flexibility, balance, and coordination.

### If I exercise a lot, do I need to eat more food or take more vitamins?

That depends largely on how much you exercise. If you're not trying to lose weight, you'll need to figure out how many calories you're burning and increase your caloric intake to meet the demand. If you exercise a great deal, you may need to increase the amount of B vitamins and others you ingest in order to provide your body with the enzymes it needs to transform the food you eat into the energy your muscles need to perform their work. However, you shouldn't assume that eating vastly more protein or taking megadoses of vitamins, minerals, or other potions would make you fitter, faster, or stronger. If you have any further questions, you should consult a qualified nutritionist who can advise you on your specific metabolic needs and how to meet them.

**My mother is getting older; she's nearly seventy-five now. Does the Food Guide Pyramid apply to her as well?**

Generally speaking, yes. However, there are some special considerations to keep in mind when it comes to creating a healthy diet for older Americans. One of the major changes in eating patterns in most people over the age of sixty-five is the need to reduce the number of calories eaten. Unless your mother is getting plenty of regular exercise, she simply won't need to eat as much food. Even if she is active, her metabolism will slow down naturally as she ages.

Another age-related change involves the senses: Most older people cannot smell or taste as well as they did in their younger days. In fact, the number of taste buds actually declines with age, and the first to go are those that detect sweet and salt. This results in most food tasting bitter and sour. Add to this the fact that medications can affect both appetite and the ability to absorb nutrients, and you can see that the stage is set for malnutrition to take hold.

Discuss with your mother her daily eating habits. If she's not taking a multivitamin or B-complex supplement already, by all means encourage her to do so starting today. As discussed in chapter 1, making sure that your mother gets all the vitamin Bs she needs can mean the difference between healthy, vital aging and sinking into depression, apathy, and dementia. (We discuss this further in chapter 7.) If she complains about being bored with her diet, try to spice it up with new foods and new flavors. If you need further help, consult a qualified nutritionist. You can probably find one through your own doctor. Finally, make sure your mother stays active; just a twenty-minute walk after dinner each night can make all the difference in the world.

## GETTING ENOUGH OF THE Bs

Now that you've gained a basic understanding of what a healthy, balanced diet looks like, it's time to see how you can choose foods from within that framework that will give you the best chances of increasing your intake of the all-important B vitamins.

### THE BEST SOURCE OF Bs

The B vitamins are most plentiful in whole grains such as wheat, rice, oats, and rye, as well as in liver and other organ meats, beef, chicken, fish, eggs, and other animal protein sources. You can also find the Bs in green leafy vegetables and some fruits, especially bananas. Here's a chart that lists the B vitamin content of some of the most common and rich sources of the vitamins:

## PLENTIFUL SUPPLIES: THE B VITAMINS IN FOOD

| FOOD | AMOUNT | B1 mg | B2 mg | Niacin mg | B5 mg | B6 mg | Folic acid mcg | Biotin mcg | B12 mcg |
| --- | --- | --- | --- | --- | --- | --- | --- | --- | --- |
| RDI | | 1.5 | 1.7 | 20 | 10 | 2.0 | 400 | 30–100 | 6.0 |
| Wheat bread | 1 slice | .11 | .07 | .9 | .2 | .05 | 14 | 0 | 0 |
| Oatmeal, cooked | 1 cup | .26 | .05 | .03 | .5 | .05 | 9 | 9 | 0 |
| Cheddar cheese | 1 ounce | .01 | .11 | .2 | .4 | .02 | 18 | 10 | .23 |
| Milk | 1 cup | .09 | .40 | .2 | .8 | .10 | 12 | 11 | .87 |
| Egg | 1 large | .04 | .14 | 0 | .9 | .06 | 24 | 20 | .66 |
| Cod, baked | 3 ounces | .08 | .07 | 2.1 | 0 | .24 | 0 | 18 | .89 |
| Brown rice | 1 cup | .20 | .02 | 2.6 | .8 | .30 | 8 | | 0 |
| Spaghetti | 1 cup | .20 | .13 | 2.3 | .2 | .13 | 0 | | 0 |
| Banana | 1 medium | .05 | .11 | .6 | .3 | .66 | 22 | 6 | 0 |
| Brewer's yeast | 1 ounce | 4.4 | 1.2 | 10.7 | 0 | 0 | 0 | 85 | 0 |
| Soybeans, cooked | 1 cup | .27 | .49 | .7 | .3 | .40 | 93 | 44 | 0 |
| Beef liver | 4 ounces | .23 | 4.60 | 12.1 | 5.2 | 1.1 | 245 | 95 | 80 |
| Chicken, white, roasted | 3.5 ounces | .07 | .12 | 12.4 | 1.0 | .60 | 1.0 | 9 | 34 |
| Peas, cooked | 1/2 cup | .04 | .07 | .6 | .5 | .05 | 51 | | 0 |

As you can see, although the amount of each nutrient is rather small in most cases, so, too, is the total amount of the B vitamins you need each day. By following the guidelines we set in the section above the Food Guide Pyramid and eating a wide variety of foods, you can certainly approach the goal of obtaining your RDIs from your diet.

### If I eat liver or another food with high levels of folic acid twice a week, but not much of the nutrient at other times, will I still run a deficit?

That's a very good question, and the answer is probably not, especially if you take a multivitamin or a B-complex supplement. Although your body doesn't store water-soluble vitamins for more than a few days, you shouldn't be so concerned about boosting your levels much over the RDI every day. Enriching your diet with healthy, vitamin B–rich food over the course of the week, and then the month, will slowly but surely increase your chances of staying healthy and rebalancing any deficiencies or excesses you've developed in the past.

### I'm trying to lose weight. Will that affect my vitamin B levels?

Yes, and in a positive way. A 1988 study in the *American Journal of Clinical Nutrition* showed that when the fat content of the typical U.S. diet was reduced from 44 percent to 25 percent of the total calories, there was actually a marked improvement in the overall nutritional content of the diet. As the amount of fat decreased, carbohydrates in the form of grains, fruits, and vegetables increased, providing an improvement in the vitamin and mineral content of the diet. In fact, there was an astounding 25 percent increase in the B vitamins, especially thiamine, riboflavin, niacin, $B_6$, $B_{12}$, and folic acid.

## How does the fortification of wheat products affect my folic acid intake?

In September of 1992, the United States Public Health Service recommended that all women of childbearing age consume 400 micrograms of folic acid to reduce their risk of having a baby afflicted with neural tube defects. (You'll read more about this in chapter 4.) The Food and Drug Administration then required folic acid to be added to specific flour, breads, and other grains. Under the terms of the new rule:

• Fortification levels will range from 0.43 milligrams to 1.4 milligrams per pound of product.

• Fortification of grain products at these levels will allow the daily intake from all sources to remain below the recommended upper limit of 1 milligram per day, which is a safe level for all ages.

• Manufacturers will be allowed to make claims on the labels that the fortified products contain folic acid and that adequate intake of the nutrient may reduce the risk of neural tube defects, which we discuss in depth in chapter 4.

This fortification process certainly helps most Americans increase their intake of folic acid, but eating fortified wheat products won't address marginal deficiencies of other B vitamins or other nutrients. It's still important to supplement your diet with a multivitamin, other supplements, and certainly by eating a healthy, nutrient-filled diet.

**I'm a vegetarian. Can I obtain all the B vitamins I need in my diet?**

If you're a vegetarian, whole grains, legumes (such as beans and peas), and leafy green vegetables are good sources of most of the B vitamins, and if you also eat eggs and/or fish, you can meet your needs pretty easily. However, if you're a vegan—meaning that you eat only foods of plant origin—you usually won't be able to obtain any $B_{12}$, which is found only in animal products. We recommend that you get what you need of this vital nutrient from a supplement.

**How does cooking affect the B vitamin content of food?**

Cooking destroys the potency of several B vitamins. If you cook all of your food, rather than eating lots of fresh green leafy vegetables and fresh fruit, you should definitely consider taking vitamin supplements. That'll help increase your B vitamin intake, but because you'll lose lots of fiber as well as nutrients by cooking your food, we suggest that you attempt to increase the amount of fresh, uncooked whole food you eat every day.

**What about irradiation and other modern techniques?**

Irradiation can destroy the bacteria, fungi, parasites, and insects that infest food products. Some of these intruders not only cause food to spoil more quickly but can leave bacteria that can cause deadly food poisoning illnesses if consumed. Certain spices have been irradiated since 1983, and some grocery stores sell irradiated fruits and vegetables and poultry.

Many experts are advocating government approval for

irradiated beef, eggs, pork, and poultry. However, some nutritionists warn that the irradiation process destroys certain important nutrients. The extent of nutrient destruction depends on the nutrients at risk, the type of food, and the irradiation dosage. For example, according to an article in a 1994 issue of *Popular Science*, chicken irradiated at approved levels loses about 9 percent of its thiamine. Other experts worry that irradiation may form toxic, possibly carcinogenic, compounds in the food.

Fortunately, experts say that widespread irradiation of food is still years away in the United States, leaving time for methods to improve and for research to reveal all the hidden dangers.

Another interesting potential source of vitamin loss is in food coloring and additives to foods and to medications. Many of these additives are in a chemical family called *hydrazines*, which can deplete vitamin $B_6$ and other vitamins. Some experts suggest that the use of food additives and coloring in the past few decades accounts for the increased incidences of PMS, carpal tunnel syndrome, and other conditions that seem to be related to vitamin $B_6$.

### Can you offer any other tips for getting more Bs in the diet?

• *Start the day right.* Regularly include a fortified breakfast cereal in your meal plan. Boost your folic acid intake by tossing berries in your cereal bowl and enjoying a glass of orange or grapefruit juice.

• *Learn to love wheat germ.* This unobtrusive, crunchy grain tossed in a salad or soup or eaten by the handful as a snack can help increase your $B_2$, $B_5$, and $B_6$ vitamin intake without having to think much about it!

• *Go for the raw.* When it comes to vegetables and fruit, the less cooking you do, the better. A raw spinach salad or a side dish of very lightly steamed asparagus can provide you with high levels of folic acid—levels that drop precipitously the more heat you use to cook them.

Now that you've gained an overview of what a healthy diet rich in B vitamins looks like, as well as learned the basics of vitamin B supplementation, it's time to take a closer look at how the B vitamins affect specific health conditions. In chapter 4, we'll explore the essential relationship between folic acid and a healthy pregnancy.

## REFERENCES FOR CHAPTER THREE

Achterberg, C; McDonnell, E; Bagby, R. "How to put the Food Guide Pyramid into practice." *Journal of the American Dietician*, 1994; 1030–1035.

Gunther, JA. "The food zappers." *Popular Science*, 1994 Jan; 244 (1): 72–77, 86.

Milnes, DB; Canfield, WK; et al. "Effect of oral folic acid supplements on zinc, copper, and iron absorption and excretions." *American Journal of Clinical Nutrition*, 1984; 39: 535–539.

# · 4 ·

# Folic Acid and a Healthy Pregnancy

The upcoming birth of a baby is a joyous event for millions of women and families every year, and there's not much that most pregnant women wouldn't do to assure the health of their growing infant. The good news is that making sure you get enough of the B vitamins—something pretty simple to do as you've just seen in chapters 2 and 3—can protect developing fetuses from some of the most common and serious birth defects.

Every year, more than 4,000 infants are born in the United States with a neural tube defect—a type of birth defect that affects the proper development of the spine and nervous system. Experts estimate that at least half of these cases are related to a deficiency of folic acid, one of the B vitamins. In this chapter, we'll discuss the connection between the health of a developing fetus and the diet of his or her mother.

## NUTRITION AND A HEALTHY BABY

It is common for women to start paying serious attention to their health and nutrition once they know they're pregnant, but by then, it might be just a little too late to prevent certain defects. According to a 1995 survey by the March of Dimes, 73 percent of women waited to see the doctor until after they thought they were pregnant. Only 26 percent had talked to their doctors about pregnancy before it happened.

This delay is risky because fetal organs begin to form within three days after the first missed menstrual period, before most women even suspect they are pregnant, and are completed by the fifty-sixth day after conception. In the first three months of pregnancy, the fertilized egg increases 2.5 million times in mass, and the risks of harm to developing tissues are far greater than during the rest of the pregnancy when the increase in mass is only 230 times. Of ultimate importance to this process are the nutrients provided to the growing fetus by the mother. The very structure of the brain is influenced by what mothers eat during pregnancy, including folic acid, vitamin $B_6$, vitamin $B_{12}$, and the cofactor, choline.

## WHO'S AT RISK

Of special concern are women who have been using birth control pills and those with poor eating habits. Both of these groups may be deficient in folic acid and the other B vitamins.

- *Birth control pills.* Oral contraceptives affect the absorption and use of several nutrients within the body, including folic acid and the other B vitamins. Scientists are unsure how long it takes after women stop using the Pill for adequate levels of nutrients to be restored, but most experts suggest taking increased doses of the B vitamins, especially, in the months leading up to and during pregnancy.

• *Poor dietary intake.* As discussed, getting all of the essential vitamins and minerals you need from your diet is tricky at best, even if you eat the right foods in the right amounts. Women in lower socioeconomic circumstances without access to fresh fruits and vegetables are at special risk for folic acid deficiency and thus at greater risk for giving birth to babies with neural tube defects.

Knowledge about the link between nutrition and birth defects, however, remains minimal. In the same 1995 survey mentioned above, the March of Dimes asked questions about nutrition. Asked what vitamins or minerals were particularly important during pregnancy, 27 percent of the women listed iron and 26 percent identified calcium, but only 6 percent mentioned folic acid. When asked about how the risk of birth defects could be reduced, most of those surveyed cited the need to avoid alcohol and cigarettes, but only 1 percent mentioned folic acid. In fact, nearly half the women questioned had never even heard of this vital mineral and only 15 percent were aware of the Public Health Service recommendation that all women of childbearing age should consume 400 micrograms of folic acid a day. The March of Dimes has since launched a $10 million campaign to educate American women on the importance of getting enough folic acid and other nutrients in their diet.

**I stopped taking the Pill about three months ago and I'm planning to get pregnant. Should I still take extra folic acid?**

Absolutely, you should. Although you may have regained the losses of nutrients caused by the depleting nature of the oral contraceptive, you'll still want to boost your intake to ensure that your new baby gets all the nutrition he or she needs in her earliest days. Remember to take a high potency multivitamin that provides you with at least 400 micrograms of folic acid every day.

**I eat a lot of fresh fruits, vegetables, and protein, and have been on the birth control pill. Will I still need to take a multivitamin before I get pregnant?**

As discussed elsewhere in this book, we think it's best for everyone to take at least a high-potency multivitamin that provides 100 percent of each essential vitamin and mineral every day to make up for the deficiencies that are almost unavoidable with today's diet. Even though you sound like you eat well, you can't be assured that the foods you eat are as rich in nutrients as they should be. Talk to your doctor. It's likely that he or she will prescribe a good prenatal vitamin for you and certainly, once you get pregnant, you'll want to boost your intake not only of the B vitamins but of other nutrients as well. We'll take that matter up later in the chapter.

## THE VITAMIN B CONNECTION

Scientists first suggested a link between neural tube defects and diet in the 1950s. The incidence of these conditions has always been higher in lower socioeconomic groups in which women typically fail to eat healthy diets. And, interestingly, babies conceived in the winter and early spring are more likely to be born with neural tube defects, perhaps because fresh fruits and vegetables are harder to find during the early weeks of pregnancy.

The connection between nutrition and the proper development of a fetus involves the need for certain nutrients in the production and division of cells and the genetic code that lies within them. Let's take a look.

## DNA: THE GENETIC CODE

The basic unit of life is the cell, an organized set of chemical reactions bounded by a membrane that protects the cell's internal structure. Our bodies are collections of trillions of cells all working together in cooperation with one another, but each having its own identity and function. Your brain cells, for instance, all cluster together to perform the intricate functions of thought, memory, and sensation. Skin cells attach to each other to cover our bodies, protecting what lies within.

With few exceptions, every cell contains all the information it needs to live and then reproduce so that the next generation of cells performs the exact same functions. The information necessary to control the chemistry of the cell is stored in a long, thin fiber called deoxyribonucleic acid, or DNA. Each bit of information along these fibers is called a gene. DNA fibers are further packaged together in structures called chromosomes.

DNA fibers are found in every cell (except mature red blood cells) and they dictate how a particular cell behaves. If the DNA within a cell becomes damaged in any way, the cell can no longer behave as it should nor can it reproduce in an appropriate way. Diseases like cancer are believed to result from the corruption of the genetic code, either through an internal malfunction or because a toxin of some kind penetrates the cell membrane and attacks the chromosome.

A new human life begins when two cells—an egg cell from the mother and a sperm cell from the father—merge to create a one-celled life form called an embryo. The embryo contains forty-six bits of genetic information—twenty-three chromosomes from the mother, and twenty-three from the father—that dictate how it will grow and even many characteristics like hair color, facial features, and intelligence.

This first cell begins to divide almost immediately, each new cell containing the information it needs to function. During the first few weeks after conception, cells that form the central nervous system—the brain and the spinal cord—gather together and start their work, and within a few days after that, cells form the heart and the blood vessels. Over the course of the next nine months or so, a whole new human being is created.

In order for these remarkable events to take place, the cells need certain nutrients in order to reproduce and perform their functions. Among the most important of these nutrients—at least when it comes to forming the cells responsible for developing the tissues of the brain and spinal cord—are folic acid and other B vitamins. As discussed in chapter 1, the B vitamins are necessary components not only of DNA but also of the cell membrane that surrounds and protects it. Folic acid seems to be particularly crucial in the process of cell division and function early in the development of an embryo.

Furthermore, recent research suggests homocysteine—
that toxic by-product of protein metabolism that plays such
a big role in the development of heart disease—may also
be a factor in neural tube defects. High levels of homocysteine may be toxic to the embryo or may affect the levels
of other important chemicals needed to create DNA. Indeed, animal studies also suggest that a decreased conversion of homocysteine to methionine could be a crucial step
in causing neural tube defects.

Finally, at least one B vitamin apparently plays another
important role in the process of DNA and cell division early
in pregnancy. Research indicates that adequate levels of
choline help to construct cell membranes, the outer sheaths
that keep cells intact. The nutrient is also a precursor molecule to the neurotransmitter acetylcholine and other chemical messengers in the brain—chemicals needed even at this
early stage of central nervous system development. Animal
studies released in 1999 found that rats fed choline-deficient
diets displayed significantly reduced rates of new cell birth,
as well as high rates of cell death, in a brain region known
as the hippocampus, which is a major neurological center for
learning and memory. The researchers conclude that the
availability of choline in the diet may be critical for the tim-
ing of cell division and migration of the cells in the developing brain.

As you can see, getting enough of the Bs through your
diet and with the help of supplements is crucial to the development of a healthy baby. Even if you're not planning
to have a baby right now, if you're of childbearing age,
make sure you obtain all the nutrients you need to stay
healthy yourself and to support a fetus if you should become pregnant unexpectedly. And if you're planning to get
pregnant in the near future, see your doctor right away. He

or she can help you create a diet, exercise, and nutrient supplement program that will maximize your chances of having a healthy pregnancy and giving birth to a healthy baby.

**I'm thinking about getting pregnant within the next year or so. When should I start taking folic acid and other B vitamins?**

That's a great question and it's terrific that you're planning ahead. According to Richard Johnston, Jr., M.D., medical director of the March of Dimes, folic acid must be consumed before conception and during the first four weeks of pregnancy in order to reduce the risks of birth defects. "Since nearly half of all pregnancies in this country are unplanned, all women capable of having a baby should be consuming folic acid every day.

**I know that some foods are now fortified with folic acid. Will the food labels tell me all I need to know about how much I'm getting per serving?**

The FDA continues to work toward ensuring that food manufacturers provide clear, accurate information on their packaging and—most importantly—to make sure that false claims about the products or their safety are not made. In order for packaging to claim that a food is "high in folic acid," it means that one serving provides 20 percent or more of the RDI for folic acid. If the label claims that the food is a "good source of folic acid," it means that one serving of it provides 10 to 19 percent of the RDI. The exact amount of folic acid available per serving is listed in the label's Nutrition Facts panel.

# NEURAL TUBE DEFECTS: THE BASICS

The neural tube is the embryonic structure that develops into the brain and spine. Every unborn baby's spine is open when it first forms, but it normally closes by the twenty-ninth day following conception. There are two major types of related neural tube defects: spina bifida and anencephaly. Anencephaly, the failure of the brain to form at all, is by far the most devastating, and babies who develop this defect miscarry, are stillborn, or die shortly after birth. Depending on its severity, spina bifida usually has a much better outcome.

## SPINA BIFIDA: AN OVERVIEW

Spina bifida is one of the most common severe birth defects in this country. Spina bifida develops when something interrupts the process of fetal development in the first few weeks after conception, preventing cells from forming the complete central nervous system, thus leaving the spinal cord exposed. If the vertebrae surrounding the spinal cord do not close properly during the first twenty-eight days after fertilization, the cord or spinal fluid bulges through, usually in the lower back.

There are two major forms of the condition. The mild form, spina bifida occulta, is only a small gap in the spine and usually causes no symptoms. According to the National Information Center for Children and Youth with Disabilities, some Americans have spina bifida occulta and don't even known they have it. The more disabling form is spina bifida aperta, which produces a noticeable sac—called a meningocele—on the infant's back that results in muscle paralysis or incontinence even after it is repaired.

In 90 percent of all spina bifida cases, a portion of the

undeveloped spinal cord itself protrudes through the spine and forms a sac protruding on the baby's back. Any portion of the spinal cord outside the vertebrae is undeveloped or damaged, causing paralysis and incontinence. The location of the sac determines how severely disabled the child will be. In general, the higher it is on the spinal column, the more paralysis there is. A large majority of babies born with spina bifida—perhaps as many as 90 percent—grow to adulthood with varying degrees of disability, including problems with bladder and bowel control, and paralysis.

## Can spina bifida and anencephaly be detected prenatally?

Spina bifida often—but not always—can be detected before birth using two or more tests. Most health care providers now routinely offer pregnant women the option of the maternal serum alpha-fetoprotein (AFP) test, a blood test taken at sixteen to eighteen weeks into the pregnancy. It measures alpha-fetoprotein, a substance produced by the fetus and secreted into the amniotic fluid, eventually entering the mother's blood. As it grows, the baby produces increased amounts of AFP until levels peak at about thirty-two weeks. Abnormally high levels of AFP may indicate that the baby has a neural tube defect, but it isn't foolproof. In about 20 percent of cases no such high levels exist, and in only 10 percent of cases of elevated levels is spina bifida present. If a woman has an elevated AFP test result, the doctor will give her a second one, followed by ultrasound.

## If the tests for spina bifida come back positive, what can be done?

Although no treatment in utero is currently available, diagnosing spina bifida during pregnancy gives parents a chance to learn all there is to know about the potential challenges they and their child will face. They can also plan to deliver their baby in a medical center equipped to treat the baby as soon as he or she is born.

## Is there treatment for spina bifida?

Doctors must repair the opening of the spine shortly after birth or the child will die. Other major surgeries often follow in the child's first years. About 85 percent of children with spina bifida develop hydrocephalus, an accumulation of cerebrospinal fluid surrounding the brain. This fluid must be drained to the abdomen or bloodstream with a surgically implanted tube. Some children with spina bifida develop foot and knee deformities caused by an interruption of spinal nerve circuits. Many patients require leg braces, crutches, and other devices to help them walk. They may have learning disabilities, and about 30 percent of children have slight to severe mental retardation, especially if they have chronic hydrocephalus. Chronic bladder and kidney problems require lifelong medical attention. Despite their need for medical attention, children with spina bifida can learn to care for many of their own needs and, with proper care, they live long and productive lives.

## Is there any way to prevent spina bifida?

Some cases of birth defects, including spina bifida, occur for no known reason. No matter how careful, how healthy, and how much a woman cares for herself and her growing baby, something can go wrong. However, as discussed, one of the best chances of preventing spina bifida apparently lies in eating a healthy diet rich in B vitamins and taking vitamin B supplements, along with getting regular exercise and avoiding toxins like alcohol and cigarette smoke. (We'll give you more tips on having a healthy pregnancy later in the chapter.)

**My sister had a baby with spina bifida. Is there a way she can protect herself from having another with the same problems?**

The U.S. Centers for Disease Control recommends that any woman who has had a baby with a neural tube defect consult her health care provider before attempting to conceive again. Her doctor will suggest that she take high doses of folic acid from the time she plans to get pregnant through the first three months of pregnancy. A 1991 British study reported that supplementation with 4 milligrams or more of folic acid before conception and through the first three months of pregnancy reduced by 70 percent the risk of neural tube defects like spina bifida in babies born to women who had already had affected babies.

## THINK AHEAD: MAXIMIZE YOUR CHANCES FOR A HEALTHY PREGNANCY

Clearly, the sooner you start planning for your baby, the better, at least when it comes to making sure that you're as healthy, fit, and well-nourished as possible. In addition to eating a balanced diet and taking vitamin supplements, you should also consider visiting your doctor for a prepregnancy checkup as soon as you think you might like to start your family. And that's especially important if you've had any problems with previous pregnancies, such as a miscarriage or preterm delivery, or if you have a chronic health problem, such as diabetes, that can increase your risk of having a baby with birth defects.

As part of your prepregnancy visit, your doctor will ask you questions about your medical history, past pregnancies, and lifestyle. You should be as open and honest with your doctor as possible, letting him or her know what medications you take, what kind of environmental exposure to chemicals or other toxins you may have, if you smoke cigarettes, and how much, if any, alcohol or recreational drugs you use. If you do smoke or drink, your doctor will admonish you to avoid such substances at all costs before, during, and—at least in the case of cigarettes—after your pregnancy. Smoking doubles the risk of ectopic pregnancy (a pregnancy that forms outside of the uterus that must be removed) and a woman who drinks heavily risks having a baby with fetal alcohol syndrome, which involves a pattern of mental and physical defects. Even light or moderate drinking can pose a risk to the fetus.

At this time, your doctor will also test you for infections, sexually transmitted diseases, and other health hazards. Blood tests will measure your immunity to infections that could cause birth defects such as mental retardation, including rubella (German measles), toxoplasmosis (a parasitic infection), hepatitis B, and chicken pox. He or she may also discuss inherited diseases that you could potentially pass on to your baby. Blood tests can identify carriers of such disorders as Tay-Sachs disease, sickle cell anemia, and thalassemia. If you do carry the potential to pass on a genetic disease, your doctor will recommend further genetic testing and counseling.

If you're seriously overweight, your doctor may well suggest that you lose some weight before you become pregnant. Two studies published in the *Journal of the American Medical Association* found that obese women are two to four times more likely to have a baby with a neural tube defect than women who are not significantly overweight.

**I work a full-time job, have two small children, and just found out I'm pregnant. Needless to say, I'm under stress. Can stress affect my pregnancy?**

Stress is only bad if you are unable to handle the challenges set before you, and you begin to feel overwhelmed or depressed. When stress begins to build to uncomfortable levels, it can be harmful for pregnant women. In the short term, high levels of stress can cause fatigue, sleeplessness, anxiety, poor appetite or overeating, and headaches and backaches. Over the long term, high stress levels can contribute to serious health problems, such as lowered resistance to infections, high blood pressure, and heart disease. Of particular interest to this book is the fact that high stress is directly related to the depletion of B vitamins, particularly of folic acid and $B_6$, which are so important to the health of your fetus. If you feel under stress while you are pregnant, then it's even more important for you to boost your intake of these essential nutrients.

Furthermore, high stress can increase the risk of a poor outcome in other ways—premature labor, low birth weight, and miscarriage. A 1993 study by researchers at the University of California found that women who reported more life-event stresses (such as a death in the family, divorce, loss of job, or financial difficulties) had a significantly increased risk of having low birth-weight babies and to deliver prematurely. It appears likely that stress increases the levels of a group of hormones that restrict blood flow to the placenta so that the fetus may not receive the nutrients and oxygen it needs for optimal growth. These same hormones also play a role in triggering labor and, therefore, increased levels of these hormones may increase the risk of preterm labor.

Other tips for reducing stress during pregnancy include:

• *Exercise.* As long as you get a clean bill of health from your doctor, exercising while pregnant can help you both maintain your sanity and your physical health. Walking, swimming, riding a stationary bicycle, and joining a pre-natal aerobics class are all excellent choices. Exercises that require jerky, bouncy movements and being outside in hot weather are not good choices. Other sports to avoid include downhill skiing, rock climbing, and horseback riding.

• *Develop a good support network.* Just being able to talk to friends and loved ones about the challenges you face can go a long way in alleviating stress, to say nothing of the joy of sharing such a remarkable experience will bring to you.

• *Practice stress reduction techniques.* Meditation, deep breathing exercises, and yoga are all excellent and safe ways for you to relax your body and mind. Your local YMCA, health spa, or your doctor can recommend classes that will introduce you to one or more of these stress-reduction methods.

### Should I change my diet when I'm pregnant?

You should follow the Food Guide Pyramid described in chapter 3 in terms of balancing your intake with the proper proportions of the main food groups, but you really are eating for two and thus must boost your caloric intake and your intake of certain nutrients for the nine months you're pregnant and for the months you breast-feed. The

March of Dimes suggest increasing your daily food portions to include:

- 6 to 11 servings of breads and other grains
- 2 to 4 servings of fruit
- 4 to 6 servings of milk and milk products
- 3 to 4 servings of meat and protein foods
- 6 to 8 glasses of water

To put it another way, the National Academy of Sciences recommends that pregnant women eat an average of 150 calories more per day in the first three months of pregnancy and 350 extra calories per day for the remaining six months. Although you'll want to monitor your weight, a total weight gain of about twenty-five to thirty pounds is usually recommended. Your weight gain should be at its lowest during the first trimester and should steadily increase through the third trimester, when the fetus and the placenta reaching their largest sizes. Interestingly, breast-feeding after you give birth will help you to drop those pounds; a woman who breast-feeds expends 600 to 800 more calories per day than one who doesn't.

**It's all well and good to say that I'm supposed to have a healthy diet, but I have such morning sickness (it's sometimes afternoon and evening sickness, too!) that I'm worried about getting enough nutrition. What can I do?**

Nausea and vomiting in early pregnancy are uncomfortable but rarely serious side effects of the momentous hormonal changes your body is going through at this time. Interestingly, you may get some much-needed help from taking some extra doses of vitamin $B_6$—about 75 milligrams taken as three divided doses, one every eight hours. Two recent studies performed at the University of Iowa found that pregnant women who took 25 milligrams of vitamin $B_6$ every eight hours experienced significantly less vomiting and nausea than women who did not take the vitamin.

No one really knows exactly why $B_6$ works to help alleviate nausea or vomiting, but the reason may lie in the involvement in $B_6$ in the production of hormones. In any case, as long as you get your doctor's permission before taking the supplements, you should try the $B_6$ solution to your morning sickness. Do not take more than the recommended dosage; taking more than 150 milligrams per day over a long period of time can damage the nerves, resulting in numbness and tingling.

Other tips to soothe your roiling stomach include:

• *Keeping meals small and thus easy to digest*

• *Drinking fluids between, but not with, meals, and thus avoiding uncomfortable bloating*

• *Avoiding foods that are greasy, fried, or highly spiced that can upset a stomach even under optimal conditions*

• *Drinking ginger tea and eating fresh ginger*

## What other tips can you give me for having a healthy baby?

The March of Dimes offers the following tips for taking care of yourself in the months before you get pregnant:

• *Immunize.* If you're not immune to chicken pox and rubella, check with your health care provider about getting vaccinated before you conceive.

• *Attain your ideal weight.* Being overweight or underweight may cause problems during your pregnancy.

• *Focus on your family tree.* If you've had problem pregnancies or birth defects in your family, you should talk to your health care provider and/or a genetic counselor when appropriate.

• *Adopt a healthy lifestyle.* Get plenty of exercise, eat a healthy, balanced diet as described here and in chapter 3, and don't drink alcohol, smoke cigarettes, or use drugs.

• *Avoid exposure to toxic substances and chemicals.* Cleaning solvents, lead and mercury, some insecticides, and paint thinners and removers all have been shown to put a developing fetus at risk.

• *Don't handle cat litter.* Cat feces can contain toxoplasmosis, an infection that can seriously harm a developing fetus.

• *Beware of medications.* Never take any medications—even over-the-counter drugs—unless you first ask your physician.

As you can see, making sure you obtain at least the RDIs for all your B vitamins can maximize your chances for having a healthy baby. But the B vitamins aren't just for women. In the next chapter, you'll see how the Bs will help you fight against the nation's number-one killer, cardiovascular disease.

# REFERENCES FOR CHAPTER FOUR

Centers for Disease Control. "Recommendations for the use of folic acid to reduce the number of cases of spina bifida and other neural tube defects." *Morbidity and Mortality Weekly Report*, 1992; 41: RR14.

Czeizel, A; Dudas, I. "Prevention of the first occurrence of neural-tube defects by preconceptual vitamin supplementation." *New England Journal of Medicine*, 1992; 327: 1832–1835.

Fenster, L; et al. "Psychological stress in the workplace and spontaneous abortion." *American Journal of Epidemiology*, 1995; 11 (142): 1176–1183.

Mills; JL; McPartlin, JM; Kirke, PN; Conley, MR; et al. "Homocysteine metabolism in pregnancies complicated by neural tube defects." *Lancet*, 1995; 345 (8943): 149–151.

Mukherjee, MD; Sandstead, HH; Ratnapark MV; et al. "Maternal zinc, iron, folic acid, and protein nutriture and outcome of human pregnancy." *American Journal of Clinical Nutrition*, 1984; 40: 496–507.

Shaw, GM; et al. "Risk of neural tube defect–affected pregnancies among obese women." *Journal of the American Medical Association*, 1996, 275 (14): 1093–1096.

Tamura, T; Goldenberg, RL; Freeberg, LE; et al. "Maternal serum folate and zinc concentrations and their relationships to pregnancy outcome. *American Journal of Clinical Nutrition*, 1992; 56: 365–370.

Wadhwa, PD; et al. "The association between prenatal stress and infant birthweight and gestational age at birth: a prospective investigation." *American Journal of Obstetrics and Gynecology*, 1993; 169 (14): 858–865.

Wald, N; Sneddon, J; Densem, J; et al. of the Medical Research Council Vitamin Study Group. "Prevention of neural tube defects." *Lancet*, 1991; 338: 131–137.

# · 5 ·
# The Bs and Your Cardiovascular Health

Did you know that cardiovascular disease remains the nation's number one killer, claiming the lives of more than 950,000 people every year, representing 41.8 percent of all deaths in this country? If you didn't realize how serious the disease remains, you're not alone. In 1997, a survey performed by the Quaker Oats Company revealed a shocking statistic: Despite decades of a massive education effort by the U.S. government and private organizations, fewer than half of Americans still do not realize that heart disease is the leading cause of death in the United States. According to the survey, 57 percent named other sources, including 28 percent who thought cancer was the leading cause of death. Yet, according to statistics compiled by the Centers for Disease Control, almost one in two Americans dies of cardiovascular disease, 500,000 of them of heart attacks.

Although there may be a genetic component to cardiovascular disease, most causes of heart attack, stroke, peripheral vascular disease, and related conditions remain under your control to prevent. One big step in the right direction is to boost your intake of the B vitamins. We'll show you in this chapter just how strong the connection is between adequate levels of folic acid, $B_6$, and $B_{12}$ and a healthy cardiovascular system. First, though, let's explore the world of blood and blood vessels.

## THE CARDIOVASCULAR SYSTEM: AN OVERVIEW

Cardiovascular disease is a blanket term that describes a wide variety of related conditions. Some involve problems with the blood vessels themselves, others with the heart (called coronary artery disease), and still others with blood components like platelets and red blood cells. Often, a problem in one area of the system has widespread effects.

In order to live, each cell of the body must have a steady supply of oxygen and other nutrients as well as a way to eliminate the waste products it produces. The human circulatory system that transports these nutrients and wastes consists of three main components: the blood itself, the vessels that carry it, and the heart. The heart, a sac of specialized muscle tissue, lies at the center of this system. Essentially a sophisticated pump, the heart rhythmically contracts about seventy-two times a minute to force the blood out through the vessels and then back to the heart.

The average adult human body contains about eleven pints of blood that the heart pumps through the body. Every time the heart beats, it sends two to three ounces of blood from its pumping chamber (the left ventricle) into the largest artery (the aorta). The large arteries that supply blood to the head, internal organs, and the arms and legs stem from the aorta; these large arteries then branch into smaller and smaller vessels, the smallest being the arterioles and capillaries. On the way back to the heart, the blood travels through veins and their smaller subset, venules. Remarkably, it only takes a minute for a drop of blood to make its way all the way through the body.

Most diseases of the cardiovascular system, including those that cause heart attacks and strokes, can be traced to the condition known as atherosclerosis. Atherosclerosis occurs when the walls of the blood vessels become scarred and then thickened by an accumulation of material, including fats and lipids. Although there are many risk factors for cardiovascular disease—and we'll discuss them all later in the chapter—when it comes to the B vitamins, there are two known processes involved:

• *Free radical damage.* As you may remember from chapter 1, free radicals are molecules in the body that have the power to damage healthy cells. Free radicals can not only directly damage blood vessel walls by attacking their cell membranes, but they also react with the fatlike substance in the blood called cholesterol, turning into a harmful material that attaches to the vessel walls. As you know, some of the B vitamins, particularly folic acid and $B_6$, have antioxidant properties that can help prevent free oxidant damage to the heart and blood vessels.

• *High homocysteine levels.* In 1995, an analysis of thirty-eight previously conducted studies published in the *Journal of the American Medical Association* confirmed that high blood levels of homocysteine were clearly associated with cardiovascular disease and that folic acid lowered levels of the amino acid. Other studies have reported that vitamins $B_6$, $B_{12}$, and choline also lower homocysteine levels.

### I've only just started hearing about homocysteine and heart disease. Is it a new discovery?

The role of homocysteine in cardiovascular disease was first proposed in 1969 by Kilmer McCully, M.D., now a pathologist at the Veterans Affairs Hospital in Providence, Rhode Island, but it has taken almost a quarter century for it to become medically acceptable. McCully reported finding arterial disease in an infant who had died from a rare metabolic defect that resulted in very high levels of homocysteine. The baby had severe arteriosclerosis, similar to the arterial disease seen in young people with a better-known genetic disorder called homocystinuria.

Homocysteine is an intermediate in the conversion of certain amino acids—methionine and cysteine—a process requiring activated folic acid, vitamin $B_6$, and vitamin $B_{12}$. Research shows that homocysteine is toxic to the lining of the blood vessels, called the vascular endothelium, but undergoes rapid enzymatic metabolism so that it is not normally present in the bloodstream. However, a surprisingly large number of people have elevated blood levels of this body chemical, some because they inherit a condition that keeps levels high and others for unknown reasons, but probably related to a deficiency of the B vitamins necessary to prevent homocysteine from collecting in the bloodstream.

Furthermore, there appears to be a relationship among homocysteine, folic acid, and $B_6$ in the narrowing of the carotid artery, which feeds blood to the head and neck, and is implicated in stroke and heart disease. According to some studies, people with high levels of homocysteine are twice as likely to suffer from clogged arteries than are people with low levels of amino acid.

## Are there other risk factors besides free radicals and high homocysteine levels?

Cardiovascular disease involves a complex constellation of symptoms and risk factors. There is never one simple cause nor one simple solution. Here is a list of the major risk factors for this common but potentially fatal group of diseases:

• *Age.* Your risk of cardiovascular disease increases as you get older. More than half of those who have heart attacks are sixty-five years or older, and four out of five of those who die of such attacks are over age sixty-five. On the other hand, a full 5 percent of heart attacks occur in people under forty, and twenty-eight percent of stroke victims are under the age of sixty-five.

• *Gender.* At all ages, men are at more risk for cardio-vascular disease than are women. After menopause (and the loss of protection from the female hormone estro-gen), however, women's rates quickly rise to nearly those of men. Both heart attacks and strokes are more deadly in women than in men, both because women are often unaware of the high risk they have of developing cardiovascular disease and because the symptoms of heart attack tend to be more subtle in women than in men.

• *High blood pressure.* Also known as hypertension, high blood pressure is the risk factor for cardiovascular disease that affects the greatest number of Americans. Estimates vary, but anywhere from 35 million to more than 60 million people have elevated blood pressure. One way that high blood pressure damages blood vessels is by increasing the inflammatory response, which brings harmful chemicals to the cell linings of blood vessels, weakening them and making them more susceptible to plaque buildup and arteriosclerosis. Hypertension often occurs together with other risk factors, particularly obesity, elevated levels of cholesterol and triglycerides, and diabetes mellitus.

Chronic, untreated high blood pressure is an important risk factor in heart disease, stroke, and peripheral vascular disease. In addition, recent research published in the American Heart Association journal *Stroke* indicates that high blood pressure speeds the loss of memory and other cognitive abilities in the elderly and actually causes their brains to shrink in size—and this problem results even in the absence of stroke.

• *High cholesterol.* As discussed, having too much of certain kinds of fat and other lipids puts you at higher risk of developing plaques that narrow the blood vessels and reduce blood flow to vital areas of the body (arteriosclerosis). Cholesterol travels through the bloodstream by combining with other lipids and certain proteins. When combined, these substances are called lipoproteins. One type of lipoprotein, called high-density lipoprotein (HDL), is beneficial to the body because it carries cholesterol away from blood vessel walls. Another type of lipoprotein, low-density lipoprotein or LDL, is considered harmful because it carries about two-thirds of circulating cholesterol to the cells.

As discussed, research indicates the LDL cholesterol may become harmful only after it has been oxidized, or combined with oxygen. Oxidation occurs primarily when the cells become damaged by free radicals, unstable molecules that enter the body through the food you eat and the air you breathe. The B-complex vitamins can both disarm free radicals and protect the cell membranes from damage by the free radicals that remain.

• *Smoking.* A smoker's risk of cardiovascular disease is more than twice that of a nonsmoker. Overall, experts estimate that 30 to 40 percent of the approximately 500,000 deaths from coronary artery disease each year can be attributed to smoking. The nicotine in cigarette smoke increases heart and vessel activity, while many of the other toxic substances contribute to the acceleration of arteriosclerosis. Cigarette smoke raises the amount of fat and cholesterol circulating in the bloodstream, which form plaque on artery walls. Carbon monoxide, another ingredient in cigarette smoke, damages the cells that form the inner linings of arterial walls, making them more susceptible to plaque buildup.

To make matters worse, carbon monoxide is carried through the bloodstream by the same blood component, hemoglobin, that transports oxygen. The more carbon monoxide in the bloodstream, the less oxygen is being carried to the vital organs, including the heart and brain. Therefore, at the same time that nicotine is stimulating heart and blood vessel activity, carbon monoxide prevents oxygen from helping the body do this extra work. Over time, this extra stress weakens both heart and vessel walls and further paves the way for arteriosclerosis and hemorrhage. Finally, cigarette smoke also causes chemical changes in the blood itself, causing it to become more viscous, or sticky, which results in the formation of large blood clots.

• *Diabetes mellitus.* Defined as an inability to properly

metabolize carbohydrates, diabetes mellitus also represents a significant risk for cardiovascular disease. Experts feel this is due in part to the fact that people with diabetes have much higher levels of fat in the bloodstream than those with healthy blood sugar metabolism. Those with type II diabetes (associated with obesity) have elevated levels of insulin, which is irritating to the lining of the arterial walls, leading to arteriosclerosis. In addition, both the small and large blood vessels of those with diabetes tend to thicken abnormally, conditions known as microangiopathy and macroangiopathy. Diabetes also may trigger the development of high blood pressure.

• *Obesity.* Being more than 20 percent over your ideal weight is a known risk factor for cardiovascular disease of all types. Even ten extra pounds places a burden on the heart and blood vessels; for each pound of excess weight, the heart is forced to pump blood through an additional several hundred extra miles of blood vessels a day. Overweight people also tend to eat too much fat and cholesterol, which contributes to the development of arteriosclerosis. Obesity and diabetes are twin threats; most people with diabetes are overweight and many overweight individuals will develop diabetes. The combination of hypertension, diabetes, and obesity often leads to heart attack and stroke.

• *Sedentary lifestyle.* It's been official since 1992: The American Heart Association now designates inactivity as one of the four top risk factors for the development of cardiovascular disease. The Centers for Disease Control in Atlanta, Georgia, estimate that about 250,000 deaths per year can be attributed to a sedentary lifestyle.

• *Stress.* Although there still isn't a proper definition for what we mean by harmful stress, there remains little doubt of a connection between unrelieved high stress and cardiovascular disease. In a recent study, for instance, performed at Duke University and published in the February 1998 issue of *New Choices: Living Even Better After 50*, stress caused a threefold higher risk of a heart attack and death in men and women with ischemia, or reduced blood flow to the heart.

Chronic stress causes blood pressure and heart rate levels to remain elevated. High levels of the stress hormone, cortisol, may lead to elevated blood sugar, platelet stickiness, and, some research shows, an increased level of blood cholesterol. All of the stress hormones have a tendency to increase free radical formation, which can lead to the oxidation of cholesterol, forming the "bad" cholesterol that damages and clogs blood vessels. Finally, chronic muscle tension can deplete the body's store of magnesium and potassium, creating an excess of calcium and sodium. The latter two minerals may act to cause vasospasm—abnormal constriction of the arteries, including the coronary arteries, which may result in a heart attack.

Furthermore, as we've discussed in previous chapters, stress depletes the B vitamins, setting your body up for an unhealthy vicious cycle. First, because the B vitamins help keep your emotions in balance by providing the brain with the raw materials it needs to process mood, thought, and movement (we'll discuss this at more length in chapter 7), they can also go a long way in relieving stress. Therefore, even a minor B vitamin deficiency can create more stress as you struggle to maintain a balance that's being challenged, which only further depletes the B vitamins. Needless to say, making sure that you obtain at least the RDIs for the Bs, and perhaps even more, whenever you enter a stressful period in your life may help alleviate your stress while keeping your heart healthy.

• *Poor diet.* A diet high in fat and cholesterol and low in antioxidants (the free radical–fighting substances contained in many fresh fruits and vegetables), contributes to the development and acceleration of cardiovascular disease.

Before we discuss what you can do to lower your risk of developing cardiovascular disease—including but not limited to boosting your intake of the B vitamins—let's take a look at the damage such disease can cause to your body.

## HEART ATTACKS

For the majority of people suffering from heart disease, the supply of oxygenated blood is reduced due to arteriosclerosis, a progressive narrowing of the open channels of the coronary arteries. As we've discussed, the buildup of plaque is a gradual process, and it may take more than twenty years before the arteries are blocked enough to produce symptoms such as shortness of breath and chest pain. If the blockage is total, a heart attack may result.

Heart attacks, also known as acute myocardial infarction, are also almost always the direct result of coronary artery disease. A blood clot or muscular spasm in a narrowed coronary vessel may suddenly block it completely, triggering an infarction (death of tissue) in the area of the heart muscle that is normally nourished by that artery. A heart attack can be dangerous because irreparable heart damage may develop within a short time after the muscle is deprived of oxygen.

## Can you describe the symptoms of a heart attack?

It's important to recognize the symptoms of a heart attack as early as possible because the earlier treatment begins, the better your chances are for a full recovery. Here's a list of the most common indications that your heart isn't receiving the oxygen it needs to survive:

- Uncomfortable pressure, fullness, squeezing, or pain in the center of the chest, lasting two minutes or longer

- Pain spreading to the shoulders, neck, or arms

- Lightheadedness, fainting, sweating, nausea, or shortness of breath

## What is angina? Is it serious?

A primary symptom of coronary artery disease is chest pain, or angina. Angina is not itself a disease but a symptom, usually of oxygen deprivation (also known as ischemia) due to arteriosclerosis. People who suffer from angina describe a feeling of discomfort or pain, often using such words as "pressure" or "heaviness." This pain is usually located in the center of the chest but may radiate to or occur only in the neck, shoulder, arm, or lower jaw. For most people, the pain almost always occurs during or after physical activity and/or emotional stress. Ischemia may occasionally occur without symptoms of angina or other discomfort, earning it the name silent ischemia. Angina is a sign that a more serious problem—a heart attack—may be developing.

## BRAIN ATTACKS: THE TRUTH ABOUT STROKE

In February 1998, the American Heart Association announced that the estimated number of Americans afflicted with a stroke each year—500,000—is too low, that at least 731,000 people are struck by "brain attacks" every year, either their first or a recurrent episode. Stroke, also referred to as cerebrovascular disease, is a disturbance in brain function—sometimes permanent—caused by either a blockage or a rupture in a vessel supplying blood to the brain.

There are two main types of stroke: hemorrhagic strokes, which account for about 20 to 25 percent of all strokes, and ischemic strokes, which account for about 70 percent of strokes. Hemorrhagic strokes involve blood seeping from a hole in a blood vessel wall into either the brain itself or the space around the brain. Most people who have hemorrhagic strokes have a history of hypertension, diabetes, and arteriosclerosis. Ischemic strokes are caused by a lack of blood flow to the brain. In some cases, oxygen deprivation is caused by a clot (thrombus) that blocks blood flow in an artery. Another kind of ischemic stroke involving a clot is called a cerebral embolism, which is caused by a wandering clot that forms in one part of the body, breaks loose, and travels in the bloodstream until it lodges in an artery in the brain or in a vessel leading to the brain. A third form is called lacunar infarctions, which are the result of the complete blockage of arterioles, the very small ends of the arteries that penetrates deep into the brain.

## PERIPHERAL VASCULAR DISEASE

Peripheral vascular disease (PVD) is essentially the same condition as coronary artery disease, which it often accompanies, and similar to the process involved in stroke. In all three conditions, plaque deposits form in arteries, decreasing their blood-carrying capacity. That causes pain during exertion because the muscles served by the clogged arteries aren't getting enough oxygen. While the pain this blockage causes is called angina when it occurs in the heart, it is called claudication when it occurs in the legs.

The symptoms of PDV are a cramping pain in the muscles of the calves, thighs, or hips during exercise. At first, the pain goes away quickly when you stop exercising. But, as the disease progresses, the pain begins earlier during exertion and becomes more severe. When the tissues become chronically starved for blood, you may experience foot pains while at rest that are worse when you elevate the foot. In its advanced stages, leg ulcers, even gangrene can set in.

## Is PVD a serious disease?

Peripheral vascular disease is not only quite painful and potentially disabling, it also is a warning sign of much more serious consequences. Consider this: A ten-year study at the University of California reported a high death rate from cardiovascular disease among patients with even mild peripheral artery blockage. For patients with severe leg artery problems, the ten-year mortality rate was as much as fifteen times that of people with no peripheral vascular disease.

Furthermore, peripheral vascular disease is the leading cause of amputations in this country. It generally strikes those over the age of forty-five and is a frequent complication of diabetes. As is true for other forms of cardiovascular disease, PDV is more likely to affect smokers, people with high blood pressure and/or high cholesterol levels, a family history of artery disease, and those who are obese.

**My sister suffers from something called Raynaud's disease. Is that a type of PVD?**

Actually, no. Raynaud's disease is a relatively rare condition, seen most commonly in women between the ages of fifteen and fifty. It is caused by an overconstriction of blood vessels in fingers, toes, and, less frequently, the ears and nose. The cause of the condition is unknown. A more common condition is called Raynaud's Syndrome, or Raynaud's Phenomenon. This is a mild constriction of the fingers and toes, sometimes associated with the digits turning white or bluish. It can occur with autoimmune diseases such as lupus and rheumatoid arthritis, or alone.

## PREVENTING AND TREATING CARDIOVASCULAR DISEASE: THE ROLE OF THE Bs

Preventing and treating heart disease means first identifying, as much as possible, your risk factors and then doing your best to eliminate or mitigate them as much as possible. That means if you're overweight, it's time to cut down on the pounds. If you lead a sedentary life, it's time to start exercising on a regular basis (as long as you have your doctor's approval). And if you're not eating enough fresh fruits and vegetables and taking a high-potency vitamin that contains 100 percent or more of the RDIs for antioxidants like vitamins C, E, and B-complex, it's time to start watching your diet and taking supplements. We'll show you the connection in this section.

**How can the B vitamins help reduce my risk for cardio-vascular disease?**

- *Reducing homocysteine levels.* Taking at least the RDI of vitamins $B_6$, $B_{12}$, choline, and folic acid will help you keep homocysteine levels low and thus avoid the damage that this toxic substance can do to the heart and vessels.

- *Protecting cell membranes.* As discussed in chapter 4, choline plays a special role in maintaining the integrity of cell membranes, including those that line the heart and vessels, thus protecting tissue from damage.

- *Lowering cholesterol.* Studies show that pantothenic acid, in particular, can lower serum cholesterol levels and improve lipid metabolism, even in patients with diabetes who have particular difficulty in this area.

**What doses of the B vitamins should I take to protect myself against developing cardiovascular disease?**

If you're healthy now, your first goal is to get at least RDIs for all of the B vitamins (see chapter 2 for more information), exercise on a regular basis, and eat a healthy, balanced diet concentrating on complex carbohydrates, fresh fruits and vegetables, and lean protein. If you have specific problem areas, such as high blood pressure or atherosclerosis, you may want to boost the levels of choline, pantothenic acid, folic acid, vitamin $B_6$, and vitamin $B_{12}$ up to three or four times their RDIs and perhaps more. The good news about these vitamins is that you'll excrete any excess, so there is no chance that you could develop a toxic reaction. On the other hand, there is little evidence that megadoses of these vitamins will provide any benefit to your health.

Do keep in mind that nutrition is a highly individual matter, and to address your particular needs—especially when it comes to a complex disorder like cardiovascular disease—may require a visit to a qualified nutritionist for more advice.

### What else can I do to bring down my cholesterol levels, which are on the high side?

The first thing you need to do is examine your diet—and not necessarily for the presence of the typical culprits like eggs and cheese. Indeed, evidence suggest that it isn't so much the quantity of dietary cholesterol you eat but rather what happens once cholesterol is in your bloodstream. If you're eating plenty of fresh fruits and vegetables that contain both antioxidants to fight against free radicals and B vitamins to lower homocysteine levels, you may be surprised how quickly you can gain control over your high-cholesterol problem.

Another relatively safe way is to take an extra daily dose of vitamin $B_3$ or niacin, which not only knocks down total cholesterol but also decreases the bad form of cholesterol. As you may remember from chapter 2, however, you've got to monitor your intake of niacin with care because the side effects can be quite disturbing and even dangerous. You should not take higher than the RDI if you have active peptic ulcers, liver disease, diabetes, or glaucoma. The other potential problem is the niacin flush—a hot, tingling, prickly sensation. As mentioned in chapter 2, your best bet is to slowly increase your intake to no more than 3,000 milligrams a day; as soon as you start feeling signs of discomfort, decrease the dose. One form of niacin, called in-osilol hexaniacinate, causes less flushing.

There are also several dietary measures you can take to lower your cholesterol levels, starting with breakfast. Research shows that only one to two ounces of oats or oat bran per day can produce significant reductions in blood cholesterol. Oatmeal, beans, peas, lentils, barley, and bananas are all good sources of B vitamins (including niacin) and other cholesterol-fighting substances. Garlic appears to have a marked effect on lowering cholesterol as well. Finally, you can also take a daily dose of psyllium, which is an ingredient in several over-the-counter laxatives. Recent studies show that regular doses of psyllium can lower cholesterol by 15 percent.

### I have diabetes plus high cholesterol. Can I take niacin to cut my cholesterol?

Talk to your doctor about it, but probably not. The levels of niacin necessary to lower cholesterol are considerably higher than the minimum RDI. The other danger, as you may remember from chapter 2, is that taking excess niacin can cause flushing. Again, your safest bet is to talk to your doctor and, in any case, take no more than 3,000 milligrams a day.

### What about antioxidants? What others should I be taking besides the B vitamins?

Concentrate on boosting your intake of vitamins C, E, and beta-carotene. In addition to scavenging free radicals, these antioxidants also help reduce platelet stickiness, aid in the breakdown of fats, help lower blood cholesterol levels, and increase the effectiveness of certain enzymes in the body.

One study on the role of antioxidants on heart disease was performed by Joann Manson, M.D., and Charles Hennekens, M.D., of Harvard Medical School and Brigham and Women's Hospital in Boston. After monitoring the diet and vitamin use of 87,000 nurses for more than a decade, the investigators found that the women whose vitamin E consumption was in the upper 20 percent had a 35 percent lower risk of heart disease—even when all other factors, like smoking, blood pressure, and cholesterol levels were taken into account. Those whose beta-carotene consumption was in the upper 20 percent had a 22 percent lower risk of heart disease.

**Are there other lifestyle changes I should make?**

Other ways you can reduce your risk of heart disease, stroke, peripheral vascular disease, and other forms of cardiovascular disease include the following:

• *Drop extra pounds.* As discussed, obesity is a major risk factor for cardiovascular disease of all types, and as many as 40 percent of all Americans are obese. Although losing weight—and keeping it off—can be very difficult, it is essential. If you want to maintain your health, you've got to maintain a healthy weight. The best way to diet, all experts agree, is to eat relatively small portions of a wide variety of foods—and to exercise!

• *Exercise your heart and muscles.* The physical benefits of exercise are almost too many to list: Your heart will be able to pump more blood and your vessels will be able to deliver more oxygen to the cells throughout the body in a more efficient manner. Over time, exercise will reduce blood cholesterol levels and decrease the ratio of "bad cholesterol" to "good cholesterol." Over the long haul, exercise also reduces blood pressure while increasing blood flow into the smallest arteries and veins, thus ensuring that every cell in the body receives proper nutrition. In addition, exercise has significant psychological and emotional benefits. People who exercise find that they not only feel better physically but also have a renewed sense of emotional well-being both during and in between exercise sessions.

• *Stop smoking.* Experts now recognize that nicotine is every bit as addictive as other narcotics and therefore extremely difficult to quit. Fortunately, there's help out there if you need it. Contact the American Heart Association, the American Lung Association, and even your local YWCA for information about stop-smoking groups in your area. You can also talk to your doctor or nutritionist about natural substances, like chlorophyll and the amino acid l-glutamine that may help you beat the habit.

Unfortunately, the people who need to stop smoking the most are the least likely to stop, says a new Mayo Clinic study of heart patients published in the March 1998 issue of *Mayo Clinic Proceedings.* Mayo researchers looked at the smoking patterns of more than 5,400 patients who had angioplasties (vessel clearing procedures) over a sixteen-year period. Of this group, 63 percent continued to smoke after their procedure, 51 percent continued to smoke even after a prior heart attack, and less than 10 percent sought help from a Mayo Clinic Nicotine Dependence Center. The study found that patients most likely to continue smoking were those who would benefit most by quitting—that is, younger patients who smoked the most and had more risk factors for cardiovascular disease.

• *Reduce stress.* Your heart and blood vessels take it the hardest when you're under constant stress and tension. Raising the blood pressure and heart rate is an essential part of the fight-or-flight response. According to a study presented by Johns Hopkins researchers at the American Heart Association's 1997 seventieth Annual Scientific Sessions, nearly one in four people suffer from depression after a heart attack, and these people are less likely to comply with their doctors' advice to modify their diets and exercise habits.

As you can see, nothing about cardiovascular disease is simple, including how to prevent it or alleviate it once it takes hold. We'd love to be able to tell you that taking extra doses of B-complex vitamins every day is all you need to do to keep your heart and blood vessels healthy, but that clearly isn't the case. We do hope you'll take the advice in this chapter and make all the changes we suggest, and that includes making sure that the B vitamins are represented in your diet and in your supplement intake.

## REFERENCES FOR CHAPTER FIVE

Bates, CJ; Powers, HJ; Thurnham, DI. "Vitamins, iron, and physical work." *Lancet*, 1989 Aug 5; 2 (8658): 313–314.
Challem, J. "The heart remedy your doctor never heard of." *Your Health*, 1994 June 14; 33 (12): 46–48.

Graedon, J; Graedon, T. "Over-the-counter cholesterol cutters." *Medical Self-Care*, 1989 Jan/Feb; 50: 22, 64.
Selhub, JS; et al. *New England Journal of Medicine*, 1995; 332: 286–291.

# · 6 ·

# The Cancer Connection

Cancer. Perhaps no other word in the medical lexicon sparks as much dread as that one, and for good reason. Today, cancer is the second leading cause of death in the United States, after heart disease. Current estimates say that 30 percent of all Americans will develop some kind of cancer in their lifetimes. The most common forms are cancer of the skin, lungs, colon, breast, prostate, urinary tract, and uterus.

The role of diet and nutrition in the prevention and treatment of cancer, including what appear to be vital roles for the B vitamins, continues today in laboratories around the world. Before we discuss how the B vitamins may work to protect you against cancer and how it can help you better manage chemotherapy treatment should you succumb to the disease, let's take a look at what cancer really is and how it takes hold in the body.

## UNDERSTANDING CANCER

Cancer is any group of cells that reproduce uncontrollably and abnormally, resulting in a growth called a malignant tumor. Abnormal cell reproduction can occur spontaneously, through some internal malfunction within the cell itself, or it can occur when the cell comes into contact with an external agent that triggers a disruption to the cell's normal activity.

As discussed in chapter 4, every cell in the body comes equipped with exact information—in the form of DNA, the genetic code—about how it is supposed to reproduce and behave in the body. It also contains information about how long it will live. Cancer begins when something fundamentally alters the cell's genetic code, blocking its ability to control growth processes. Cancer cells therefore continue to divide without internal restraint. In addition, cancer cells do not die at a normal rate; in fact, they die only if they outgrow their blood supply. A tumor can thus develop. In addition to encroaching on the healthy tissue from which it arises, some cancer cells may travel from the original site to another part of the body, a process called metastasis.

All cancers begin with the corruption of a single cell. When that cell divides, there are two cancer cells, when they both divide, four cancer cells, and so on. Different cancer cells divide at various rates. The time it takes for a particular cancer to double in size is called its *doubling time*. Fast-growing cancers may double in size over one to four weeks, while a slow-growing cancer may take up to five years to double. When a tumor is large enough to be seen on an X ray, it usually has to be about one-half inch in diameter. At this size, it will contain about a billion cells. Until a malignant tumor has disrupted the function of a vital cell or otherwise produces symptoms, the person whose cells have gone awry may have no idea that he or she is ill.

## What causes cancer?

The quest to identify the cause or causes of cancer continues in laboratories and research labs around the world—and the role of the B vitamins and other nutrients is often the focus of that quest. We'll discuss that role later in the chapter, but for now it's important for you to gain an understanding of some of the theories about how cancer begins and progresses:

• *Free radical damage and other carcinogens.* Scientists estimate that as many as 80 to 90 percent of all cancers may be related to environmental substances that, once in the body, attack the cells and alter the DNA, triggering cancer development. The best know carcinogens are tobacco smoke, radiation, industrial agents, and toxic substances like asbestos. Included in this group are free radicals, those unstable molecules that damage healthy cells by "stealing" particles from them. Free radical damage often causes fundamental changes in the cells' genetic material. One result of these genetic alterations may be to turn a healthy cell, one that knows how often and for how long to reproduce, into a cancer cell that grows uncontrollably.

• *Dietary influences.* More and more evidence links a healthy, nutritious diet and nutrient supplementation to the prevention of cancer. The evidence is so convincing, in fact, that the National Cancer Institute—along with other major health organizations—now recommends that all Americans eat at least five servings of fresh fruits and vegetables a day. And that's because these foods, in particular, contain high levels of antioxidants like vitamins A, C, and E and folic acid. In addition, more and more research suggests that other B vitamins—also found in fresh fruits and vegetables and in protein—may help protect against cancer in other ways.

• *Hormone imbalances.* The amount of sex hormones—estrogen in women, testosterone in men—that one is exposed to over a lifetime may play a role in the development of some cancers. Many cases of breast cancer and endometrial cancer, for instance, are related to how much estrogen the organ is exposed to during a woman's lifetime. Prostate cancer in men also appears to be affected by hormone levels.

• *Weaknesses in the immune system.* Your immune system, which consists of specialized groups of disease-fighting cells, also plays a role in protecting against cancer development. Researchers believe that many cancer cells are intercepted and destroyed by the immune system before they form tumors. If the immune system is somehow weakened, however, such interceptions cannot be made, and cancer cells are allowed to live and reproduce.

## How might the B vitamins affect cancer or cancer prevention?

That's the question more and more doctors and researchers are asking themselves today, and they're coming up with some intriguing answers. In fact, it appears that the B vitamins may help protect against every cancer-causing process.

• *Antioxidant protection.* We've already discussed the antioxidant qualities of the B vitamins. Although not as powerful as other vitamins (especially C, E, and beta-carotene) in this area, the B vitamins are able to disarm free radicals that would otherwise attack cells and corrupt the DNA within.

• *DNA synthesis and repair.* Virtually all of the B vitamins play a role in the synthesis and repair of DNA, thus maintaining the genetic code of cells and regulating normal cell division and growth. Without enough of these nutrients, then, the chances that an internal or external factor can corrupt the cell increase dramatically. In particular, folic acid plays a role in the production of S-adenosylmethionine (SAMe) that helps block DNA abnormalities.

• *Immune system booster.* Evidence exists to suggest that certain of the B vitamins may help bolster the immune system and thus help the body itself fight against cancer. A variety of research studies and anecdotal evidence indicates that all of the B vitamins—particularly $B_2$, pantothenic acid, and folic acid—play important roles in the production of several classes of immune system cells. That includes antibodies, the white blood cells that attach to and then destroy cells they consider foreign to the body, such as cancer cells.

• *Cell membrane protector.* As mentioned in previous chapters, choline, biotin, and other B vitamins help maintain the integrity of cell membranes, which may protect the DNA within the cells from damage.

What does this information mean to the development of specific cancers? Later in the chapter, we'll discuss in depth the two types of cancer for which the role of the B vitamins is best documented, colon cancer and cervical cancer. For now, here's what we know about B vitamins and the development of cancer:

- *Prostate cancer.* Prostate cancer is influenced by the presence of androgens, male hormones like testosterone. A 1999 study published in the *Journal of the National Cancer Institute* shows that antioxidant vitamins may act to prevent the androgens from binding to and then altering the internal mechanisms of prostate cells.

- *Liver cancer.* Animal studies indicate a unique role for choline in the development of liver cancer; a choline-deficient diet appears to alter the balance of cell growth and cell death in liver cells and thus promotes the survival of cells capable of becoming cancer cells.

- *Breast cancer.* A long-term study of 88,756 women (called the Nurses' Health Study) found that high daily intake of folic acid—about 600 micrograms per day—protects women who drink alcohol from developing breast cancer. According to previous research, a woman's lifetime risk for breast cancer rises 9 percent with every 10 grams/day increase in alcohol consumption. One reason could be that alcohol interferes with several aspects of the way the body metabolizes and transports folic acid, thus depleting the body of this important nutrient. Supplementing the diet with extra folic acid mitigates this problem.

- *Lung cancer.* In one recent study, Japanese doctors found that folic acid and vitamin $B_{12}$ provided protection for smokers who took 10 to 20 milligrams of folic acid and 750 micrograms of $B_{12}$ daily. These smokers experienced significant reductions in the number of potentially precancerous cells found in abnormal spots in the passageways of their lungs. Within a year, 70 percent of initially abnormal spots were reclassified as normal, and no spot had grown. In a control group, on the other hand, 77 spots remained the same, 5 percent worsened, and 18 percent got better.

### Aren't some cancers considered hereditary?

Without question, certain types of cancers run in families, which means that a genetic component is involved. Scientists have identified a type of gene, called an oncogene, that act to transform healthy cells into cancer cells if triggered by certain agents. The DNA abnormalities that lead to the development of cancer may occur in either of two types of genes—oncogenes that promote cell growth and suppressor genes that suppress cell growth. If suppressor genes are unable to do their job properly or are missing, oncogenes may be more easily triggered to begin the cancer development process. In the end, however, it probably takes "hits" from triggers like free radicals or chemicals in the environment to turn on the oncogenes or turn off the suppressor cells. That means that it's especially important to give your body the weapons it needs in the form of antioxidants and B vitamins to fight against those attackers.

## COLON CANCER

Cancer of the colon is the one of the most common and deadly cancers in the country today. Roughly 150,000 people develop colon cancer and 60,000 die from it every year in the United States. An individual has about a one in twenty lifetime risk of developing colon cancer. Although this type of cancer is highly treatable when detected early, many people delay seeking medical attention, even when there are symptoms.

The colon is part of the body's digestive system that removes nutrients from the foods eaten and stores the waste until it passes out of the body. The digestive system is made up of the esophagus, stomach, and the small and large intestines. The last six feet of intestine is called the large bowel or colon. Cancer of the colon begins when cells that line the colon become abnormal.

There are several known risk factors for this type of cancer, including:

- *Genetics.* Those with a family history of polyps and cancer of any type, but especially of the colon and of the breast, are more susceptible.

- *Age.* Most—97 percent, in fact—of all cases of colon cancer occur in men and women over the age of forty.

- *History of Crohn's disease and ulcerative colitis.* These two disorders of the gastrointestinal tract leave the cells of the colon vulnerable to damage and corruption by cancer-causing agents.

- *Poor dietary habits.* Eating a high-fat, low-fiber diet appears to be a contributing factor to the development of colon cancer.

If detected early, colon cancer is highly treatable. Screening for colon cancer includes the following methods:

- *Digital rectal exam.* A doctor inserts a gloved finger into the rectum to feel for abnormal tissue.

• *Fecal occult blood test.* This is a laboratory examination of stool for the presence of blood.

• *Sigmoidoscopy, colonoscopy, barium enema.* These are three more invasive but highly efficient ways to examine the inside of the colon.

The American Cancer Society recommends that all men and women over the age of fifty undergo regular screening for colon cancer.

## What are the symptoms of colon cancer?

That's a good question, and we hope you keep the answer in mind, because recognizing the signs that something in the digestive tract has gone awry and seeking treatment for it right away can mean the difference between life and death. The following symptoms should prompt an immediate call to your doctor:

• *Rectal bleeding*

• *Altered bowel habits*

• *Chronic abdominal cramps or pain*

• *Microscopic amounts of blood in the stool*

• *Unexplained anemia*

• *Unexplained weight loss*

It's important to understand that often there are no symptoms of colon cancer at all, which is why it's so important to receive checkups and regular screenings for the disease from your doctor.

## What exactly is a polyp, and is it always going to become cancerous?

A polyp is a growth that occurs in the colon and other organs. It is shaped like a mushroom and occurs inside the lining of the colon. It can be as small as a tiny pea or larger than a plum. It is important to note that while colon polyps start out as benign tumors, some polyps eventually become malignant. In fact, the larger the polyp, the more likely it is to contain cancer cells.

## What about the B vitamins? What's the connection there?

In the Nurses' Health Study, researchers found that women who used multivitamins containing folic acid had markedly lower cancer rates after ten years than women who did not use such supplements. And that was after they controlled for all other known risk factors (age, family history of colon cancer, aspirin use, smoking, body weight, physical activity, and intake of red meat, alcohol, and fiber).

## My father died of colon cancer. Does that mean I'm doomed to get the disease as well?

Not at all. There are plenty of steps you can take to protect yourself, including increasing your intake of the B vitamins, particularly of folic acid. Other tips for reducing your risks for colon cancer—and, in fact, most other cancers as well—include:

- *Boost your fiber intake.* In the bowel, fiber bulks up the stool, increases acidity, and reduces the concentration of potential cancer-causing agents. Although most experts recommend a daily fiber intake of 20 to 35 grams a day (about the amount in a bowl of high-fiber cereal, a serving of beans, three slices of whole grain bread, four servings of fresh vegetables, and three pieces of fruit), most Americans don't even eat half that much.

• *Boost your calcium intake.* Calcium may protect against colon cancer by binding with cancer-promoting fats and bile acids, the digestive fluid secreted by the liver. By doing so, calcium neutralizes their toxic effects and causes them to be excreted without harming the cells that line the colon.

• *Lower your fat intake.* A diet high in fat increases your chances of developing several different cancers, including breast cancer and colon cancer. Try to reduce your intake of fat to less than 25 percent of your total caloric intake, and concentrate on the monounsaturated fats found in olive oil, canola oil, and avocados.

• *Eat your green vegetables.* In addition to providing lots of B vitamins and antioxidants, green vegetables like broccoli, kale, spinach, and watercress contain other substances that can help protect against cancer.

• *Stop smoking.* Smoking raises the risk of all types of cancer, including cancer of the colon.

• *Exercise.* Exercise speeds up the rate at which food and waste pass through the digestive system, which reduces the amount of time potential carcinogens come into contact with the intestines. Exercise also increases oxygenation to healthy cells.

## CERVICAL DYSPLASIA AND CERVICAL CANCER

Every year, about 15,700 new cases of cervical cancer are diagnosed in the United States and nearly 5,000 American women die of the disease. As is true for colon cancer, most all cases of cervical cancer are curable if caught and treated early enough.

The cervix is the lower portion of the uterus that opens into the vagina. The opening allows blood to flow out of the uterus during menstruation and widens during childbirth to allow a baby to pass from the uterus through the vagina. Cervical dysplasia is a premalignant or precancerous change to the cells of the cervix that can, if left untreated, lead to cervical cancer.

One of the most common and significant risk factors for both cervical dysplasia and cervical cancer is infection with the human papilloma virus (HPV). There are more than sixty types of HPV. Types 1, 3, and 5 can cause warts on the hands and feet of children. Types 6 and 11 can cause warts on men's and women's genital areas. Other types may not cause warts but can cause changes to the cells of the vagina or cervix, including dysplasia. Indeed, HPV is the most frequent cause of cervical dysplasia.

The B vitamins, and folic acid in particular, have been found to protect the cells of the cervix, especially in women who take birth control pills. Low levels of the vitamins appear to set the stage for abnormal cell changes to take place, and experts believe that boosting intake can help prevent some cases of cervical dysplasia from developing. In addition, women who take birth control pills and have cervical dysplasia may be able to improve the health of the cervical cells by taking 10 milligrams or more of folic acid (along with a B-complex supplement).

## What exactly is a Pap test?

The Pap smear was developed in the 1940s by Dr. George Papanicolaou. Doctors perform it during a pelvic examination by scraping the entire surface of the cervix with a wooden spatula, brush, or cotton swab. Microscopic analysis of the cervical cells is then performed in a laboratory. Although it is not infallible, this test detects 95 percent of cervical cancers, and detects them at a stage when they cannot yet be seen with the naked eye. Occasionally, the Pap smear will identify an endometrial or ovarian cancer.

If you receive a negative result of a Pap smear, it means your cervix is normal. A positive result indicates the presence of some abnormal cells. It does not mean that you have cancer or even dysplasia, but it usually does mean you should undergo further examination and evaluation.

## How serious is cervical dysplasia?

With early identification and treatment, and then consistent follow-up, nearly all cervical dysplasia can be cured. Without treatment, however, about 30 to 50 percent of cervical dysplasia may progress to invasive cancer.

## Is sexual contact the only way to get HPV?

As far we know, yes. HPV is one of the most common and contagious of the sexually transmitted diseases. Even condoms may not be able to protect against it. HPV is found on all of the genital tissues, and a condom on the penis will usually not prevent its transmission. Avoiding exposure by limiting the number of sex partners is the best way to avoid this disease.

**Are there any other risk factors for cervical dysplasia and cervical cancer besides HPV?**

Cigarette smoking has also been linked to this disease. Women who smoke concentrate the chemicals nicotine and cotinine into their cervix, which harms the cells. Having multiple sex partners, especially from a young age, also contributes to the development of the disease, not only because it exposes you to more venereal diseases but to other organisms and trauma as well. If your mother took a synthetic estrogen called DES while she was pregnant with you, you're at increased risk for cervical dysplasia and cervical cancer and should be under a doctor's careful watch.

**How is cervical dysplasia treated?**

When a Pap smear reveals cervical dysplasia, the doctor usually repeats the test to confirm the results. If abnormal cells are present, the doctor may perform a procedure called a colposcopy. The colposcopy magnifies and focuses an intense light on the cervix, allowing the doctor to examine it in great detail as well as to remove a small sample of tissue for analysis. If the biopsy shows that abnormal cell growth extends into the cervical canal, a cone-shaped piece of tissue may by removed (called a cone biopsy). Removal of all dysplastic cells usually occurs next. This is done by cauterization, cryosurgery, or laser surgery. Frequent Pap smears are usually recommended to evaluate if the treatment was successful.

**How can I protect against cervical dysplasia and cervical cancer?**

First of all, make sure you're eating a healthy diet and supplementing that diet with antioxidant and vitamin B-complex supplements. By doing so, you're providing your body with the raw materials it needs to protect your cells against corruption from cancer-causing agents. Here are some other tips:

- *Have regular Pap smears.* Pap smears detect abnormal cell changes 95 percent of the time, and the earlier these cells are identified and treatment initiated, the better the prognosis.

- *Don't smoke.* Smoking is a known risk factor, not only for cervical cancer and a wide range of other cancers, but also for heart disease, stroke, emphysema, and other conditions.

- *Limit the number of sex partners, and protect yourself.* The more sex partners you have, the more likely it is that you'll get a sexually transmitted disease, which increases your risk for cervical dysplasia and cervical cancer. In addition, use barrier forms of birth control such as condoms, diaphragms, or cervical caps for further protection.

## THE ROLE OF THE Bs IN CHEMOTHERAPY SUPPORT

Chemotherapy is a common treatment for many cancers. Unfortunately, during the process of eliminating cancer cells, these powerful drugs also damage healthy cells, causing many side effects. The B vitamins can help mitigate many of these side effects. Let's take a look:

- *Malabsorption and weight loss.* Cancer often causes malnutrition and specific vitamin and protein deficiencies.

Chemotherapy also causes deficiencies by promoting anorexia, stomatitis, and alimentary tract disturbances. Deficiencies of vitamins $B_1$, $B_2$, and K and of niacin, and folic acid may also result from chemotherapy.

• *Heart damage.* Animal studies indicate that, under certain circumstances, vitamin $B_2$ (riboflavin), supplementation can help protect the heart against damage from Adriamycin, a drug used to treat several different types of cancer.

• *Skin damage.* A drug called fluorouracil sometimes causes problems on the skin of the palms of the hands and soles of the feet. Reports have appeared that 100 milligrams per day of vitamin $B_6$ can sometimes eliminate the pain associated with this condition.

We hope you can see how useful the B vitamins can be when it comes to both preventing and treating cancer. If you follow the tips in this chapter—by taking supplements of the Bs, other antioxidants, and minerals like calcium; eating a diet rich in fiber and calcium; and getting plenty of regular exercise—you'll go a long way in protecting yourself from this all too common, all too often deadly disease. In the next chapter, we'll examine the fascinating connection between the B vitamins and the way your brain and nervous system work.

## REFERENCES FOR CHAPTER SIX

Albright, CD; Liu, R; Mar, MH; et al. "Diet, apoptosis, and carcinogenesis." *Advanced Experimental Biology*, 1997; 422: 97–107.

Block, G; "The data support a role for antioxidants in reducing cancer risk." *Nutrition Review*, 1992; 56: 173–176.

Bostick, R; Potter, J; McKenzie, D; et al. "Reduced risk of colon cancer with high intake of vitamin E. The Iowa Women's Health Study." *Cancer Research*, 1993; 53: 4230–4237.

Butterworth, CE; et al. "Folate deficiency and cervical dysplasia." *Journal of the American Medical Association*, 1992; 267: 528–533.

Christensen, D. "Folic acid in multivitamins may lower colon cancer risk." *Medical Tribune*, 1998; 39 (18): 1, 5.

Dreizen, S; McCredie, KB; Keating, MJ; Andersson, BS. "Nutritional deficiencies in patients receiving cancer chemotherapy." *Postgraduate Medicine*, 1990 Jan; 87 (1): 163–167, 170.

Giovannuci, E; Stampfer MJ; Colditz, GA; Hunter, DJ; et al. "Multivitamin use, folate, and colon cancer in the Nurses' Health Study." *Annals of Internal Medicine*, 1998; 129 (7): 517–524.

Greenberg, E: Baron, J; Tosteson, T; et al. "A clinical trial of antioxidant vitamins to prevent colorectal adenoma." *New England Journal of Medicine*, 1994; 331: 141–147.

Lupulescu, A. "The role of vitamins A, beta carotene, E, and C in cancer cell biology." *International Journal of Vitamin Nutrition*, 1994; 3–14.

Mason, JB; Levesque, T. "Folate: effects on carcinogenesis and the potential for cancer chemoprevention." *Oncology*, 1996; 10: 1727–1736, 1742–1743.

Ogura, R; Humon, Y; Yoon, S. "Antioxidative effect of $B_2$ in cardiac mitochondria affected with Adriamycin." *Journal of Molecular Cell Cancer*, 1985; 17: R48.

Vukelja, SJ; Lomabardo, F; et al. "Pyroxidine for the palmar-plantar erthyrodyseshesia syndrome." *Annals of Internal Medicine*, 1989; 111: 688–689.

Wilding, G; et al. "Antioxidant vitamins inhibit role of androgens in prostate cancer development." *Journal of the National Cancer Institute*, 1999; 91: 1227–1232.

Zhang, S; et al. "Folate reduces breast cancer in drinkers." *Journal of the American Medical Association*, 1999; 281: 1632–1637.

# · 7 ·

# The B Vitamins and the Nervous System

From the moment you were conceived, your brain and nervous system have depended on the presence of the B vitamins for their growth, development, and continued vitality. They have played a role in the way your brain and nerve cells formed while you were still in the womb and have since helped to maintain the tissue as well as to produce the chemicals called neurotransmitters that allow thought, emotion, and memory to occur.

The B vitamins have a long history as antistress nutrients and mood enhancers, and for good reason. They are absolutely essential to the proper functioning of the brain and nervous system. A remarkable study in the *British Journal of Psychiatry* showed that 53 percent of psychiatric patients admitted to a hospital were deficient in at least one of the following: $B_6$, thiamine, or riboflavin. Other studies have proven that by boosting levels of these important vitamins, the brain and the mood can work better, improving such conditions as Alzheimer's disease, obsessive-compulsive disorder, depression, and even schizophrenia.

In this chapter, we'll discuss some of the two most common nervous system disorders that the B vitamins affect, Alzheimer's disease and depression, as well as examine the way that alcohol—and especially chronic alcohol abuse—affects the brain and the need for B vitamin intake. But first, let's explore the intricate world of the central nervous system and how it works.

## HOW THE BRAIN WORKS

The brain, a jellylike mass of gray tissue, is both a supercomputer and a complex chemical factory. Brain cells produce electrical signals that travel along pathways known as circuits. These circuits receive, process, store, and retrieve information, and they depend on the proper activity and balance of a variety of chemical substances known as neurotransmitters to do their jobs. The brain is the master control center of the body. Not only is it responsible for receiving and processing information from the outside world, but it also works with other systems in the body to regulate all body activities, cognitive functions, and emotional responses.

Different brain cells—and indeed all of the nerve cells throughout the body—have a unique communication system. Each neuron (brain cell) consists of a cell body with a number of fibers extending from it. The neuron communicates its message to other nerve cells by sending information out of its cell body through one of its hairlike fibers, an extension called the axon. All of the other fibers extending from the cell body, called dendrites, receive information from other cells.

The neuron is the functional unit of the brain. It receives

information, in the form of electrical impulses, at its dendrites. The impulse first passes through its cell body, then out its axon to other neurons. The axon typically divides into a number of small fibers that end in terminals, each of which forms what is called a synapse with another cell. The synapse is actually a space between the axon terminal of one neuron and the dendrite receptor of another.

Just as a car requires oil to allow its gears to shift properly, nerve cells need certain chemicals in order for this intricate circuitry to function properly. These chemicals, called neurotransmitters, trigger the connection between the axon of one neuron and the dendrite of another. Without the presence of neurotransmitters, neurons cannot send appropriate messages to other parts of the brain. In fact, the synaptic transmission is crucial to every body and mind action and reaction. The human brain, composed of more than 100 billion neurons, has at least 10 trillion synapses within it.

Brain cells produce as many as fifteen different chemicals that are used as neurotransmitters. Four of them—acetylcholine, dopamine, norepinephrine, and serotonin—are especially important to the regulation of brain activity. Indeed, vital aspects of our mental, emotional, and physical health are profoundly affected by the way in which these chemicals work with each other to keep the body and spirit in a state of flexible balance. When any part of this system becomes disturbed, physical or emotional illness may result.

**How does the brain process emotions?**

Located on top of the brain stem and buried under the cerebral cortex is a set of structures called the limbic system. Scientists believe that this highly complex and still largely unmapped region is home base to our emotions. It receives and regulates emotional information and helps govern sexual desire, appetite, and stress. Three main centers of the limbic system are the thalamus-hypothalamus, the hippocampus, and the amygdala. The thalamus-hypothalamus forms a kind of brain within a brain, regulating a variety of processes, including appetite, thirst, sleep, and certain aspects of mood and behavior. The hippocampus and the amygdala help create memory as well as gauge emotions.

What disturbs normal functioning of the brain—what makes one part of the brain more active or inactive than usual—can usually be traced to an imbalance of neurotransmitters, the nervous system's chemical messengers. An imbalance of three neurotransmitters—serotonin, norepinephrine, and dopamine—appears to be involved in most cases of depression. These same imbalances also occur in people who suffer from anxiety, eating disorders, obsessive-compulsive disorder, and several other psychological disturbances. In addition, nerve messages of all kinds—including those involved in mood, memory, thought, and movement—depend on the presence of acetylcholine, which provides the energy for synaptic transmission.

When it comes to mood, serotonin is the neurotransmitter scientists focus on the most. With the most extensive network of any neurotransmitter except acetylcholine, serotonin influences a wide range of brain activities, including mood, behavior, movement, pain, sexual activity, appetite, hormone secretion, and heart rate. People with depression have been found to have lower amounts than usual of serotonin in the brain.

Dopamine is another neurotransmitter important in the disease of depression. It follows two main pathways in the brain. One pathway connects to a portion of the brain called the corpus striatum, which controls movement. When this pathway malfunctions, as it does in such disorders as Parkinson's disease and Huntington's chorea, problems with muscle control arise. The other pathway connects to the limbic system. When dopamine does not exist in proper amounts or is unable to reach organs of the limbic system, emotional problems such as depression may occur. Norepinephrine is the third neurotransmitter thought to be involved in depression. Lower than normal amounts of norepinephrine have been measured in people who are depressed.

## How do the B vitamins affect the brain and emotions?

We cannot stress enough the importance of all eight of the B vitamins and their cofactors to the health and vitality of the brain and thus to mental and emotional well-being. Just take a look at the variety of functions these vital nutrients perform within the central nervous system:

- *Production and synthesis of neurotransmitters, particularly acetylcholine, serotonin, and dopamine*

- *Maintenance of nerve tissue in the brain and throughout the nervous system*

- *Production of myelin, the fatty substance that covers nerve cells, allowing transmission of electrical impulses to occur*

- *Production of healthy red blood cells that carry oxygen to all of the cells of the body, including the brain*

If inadequate oxygen reaches the brain for any reason, emotional and mental problems can ensue.

• *Lowering of homocysteine.* Homocysteine, the same potentially toxic body chemical responsible for many cases of heart disease and other degenerative conditions, is also linked to Alzheimer's disease and other mental and emotional disorders. A deficiency of the B vitamins—particularly of vitamin $B_6$, $B_{12}$, and folic acid—sets the stage for excess homocysteine to collect in the bloodstream and damage tissues throughout the body.

The 1990s was dubbed the Decade of the Brain because of the advances we've made in understanding the organ's anatomy and physiology, as well as in the development of the scientific tools necessary to study the tiny, intricate workings of the central nervous system. Among the strides we've made is in understanding brain disorders such as Alzheimer's disease, depression, and alcoholism. Let's take a look first at the ravages alcohol abuse does on the brain and how the B vitamins can help restore some order and health.

## ALCOHOL, THE BRAIN, AND THE Bs

To drink or not to drink . . . that has been one of the more interesting dilemmas in health care in recent years. So far, the evidence suggests that a moderate amount of alcohol—about two ounces of liquor per day—may benefit the cardiovascular system, reducing the risk of heart attack and stroke, without undermining the body's ability to store and use nutrients.

However, excessive drinking, which is more than two drinks per day, can lead to a variety of health and social conditions. In fact, according to the U.S. Department of Health and Human Services, alcohol-related problems are responsible for more than 100,000 deaths each year and cost society far more than the use of all other drugs combined—an estimated $98 billion a year. The health conditions related to excessive alcohol intake include damage to the liver, brain, and pancreas, as well as to breast cancer and osteoporosis in women.

In essence, alcohol hinders your body's ability to absorb, process, use, and store the nutrients in food. Not only are alcoholic beverages completely empty of vitamins and minerals, they also have a direct, toxic effect on the gastrointestinal tract. The result is that most of the vitamins and minerals extracted from food during digestion cannot be absorbed through the intestinal wall into the bloodstream. In addition, alcohol damages the liver, which is the organ responsible for processing nutrients; in most cases, the liver either stores the nutrients it receives or it sends them into the bloodstream after processing. The result is the slow but steady deterioration of nerve, muscle, and brain tissue that depend on the presence of these nutrients for their survival.

However, once excessive alcohol damages the liver, the body's ability to use vitamins is significantly reduced. In particular, the liver is no longer able to process, store, or use many of the water-soluble B vitamins, particularly thiamin, $B_6$, and folate. It also has trouble breaking down the fat-soluble vitamins like A, D, and E, leading to further deficiencies, and in producing the proteins necessary to transport minerals through the body, which can lead to toxic buildups of minerals in the liver.

**First of all, how do you define excess alcohol intake or alcoholism?**

Generally speaking, drinking more than one or two drinks a day is considered excessive. Alcoholism is, of course, another matter. Many people cannot tolerate any amount of alcohol without suffering the consequences of addiction, and for those people, even one drink is one too many. Some people who have a problem with alcohol lose control of their emotional and personal lives even after just a drink or two; for them, the physical problems related to alcoholism may not arise—at least not for many years. Alcoholics who drink excessively and chronically, however, risk developing several severe medical conditions, including but not limited to the problems we describe here.

**Exactly how does excessive alcohol intake cause vitamin B deficiencies?**

Excessive alcohol consumption may contribute to B vitamin deficiency in several ways:

- *Reduced intake of nutrients because of poor eating habits*

- *Impaired vitamin absorption because of alcohol-induced damage to the intestines*

- *Decreased production of enzymes necessary for vitamin metabolism*

**Are there specific conditions related to vitamin B deficiency caused by alcoholism?**

As discussed, the brain appears to be particularly susceptible to vitamin B deficiencies, particularly when it comes to vitamin $B_1$, or thiamin. Heavy drinkers are at higher risk for any of a number of emotional, mental, and nervous system conditions, including anxiety, depression, gait problems, and confusion. One disorder directly related to chronic and severe thiamin deficiency caused by alcoholism is Wernicke-Korsakoff syndrome (WKS). The acute neurological features of WKS often can be partly or completely reversed by thiamin administration along with abstention from alcohol.

## How are alcohol-related brain conditions like WKS treated?

Depending on the severity of the symptoms and the diagnosis of any other underlying conditions, doctors will often start with bolstering vitamin B-complex intake. Some doctors will prescribe 50 milligrams of thiamin a day to temporarily supplement the diets of alcoholics, but it is not known whether this can reverse the brain damage caused by a thiamin deficiency. There is a special relationship between alcohol and vitamin $B_6$, which is a nutrient we need in order for nerve impulses to travel properly from the brain to other parts of the body. Alcohol appears to destroy $B_6$; more than 50 percent of those who drink excessively seem to have deficiencies. As a result, they can shake, have an unsteady gait, or—if the deficiency is severe—suffer convulsive seizures. Luckily, eating a well-balanced diet that includes at least 2 milligrams of $B_6$ can correct the problem, as long as no more alcohol is consumed.

## Will taking more vitamins help someone stop drinking?

Unfortunately, no. There is no nutrient that will reduce the craving for alcohol and, for a person addicted to alcohol, it appears that the only cure for the disease is abstinence. Furthermore, taking vitamin and mineral supplements won't help stave off disease and deficiency as long you keep drinking. Your liver simply won't be able to process them. The good news is that after you've stopped drinking, a lot of the damage is reversible once you're on a regular, balanced diet and supplement program.

## ALZHEIMER'S DISEASE AND OTHER DEMENTIAS

The most common dementia of aging, Alzheimer's disease (AD) is a progressive disorder that primarily affects the cerebral cortex, the cap of deeply grooved tissue in which scientists believe the brain's higher powers of cognition and memory are stored. It occurs when brain tissue is destroyed, forming neurofibrillary tangles and plaques made up of a toxic protein called beta-amyloid. Research on the cause of AD continues, but no one knows for sure what triggers the destruction of brain tissue. Among the several possible causes are genetic factors (AD tends to run in families), toxic exposures, abnormal protein production, viruses, and abnormalities in the barrier between the blood and the brain. Among the toxic substances under investigation as having a role in the destruction of brain tissue is homocysteine, the by-product of protein metabolism.

### Who is at most risk for Alzheimer's disease?

AD is a disease of aging, as are other conditions that involve loss of memory and mental confusion. About 15 percent of older people eventually do develop dementia, an organic brain disorder that interferes with their mental functions and that tends to grow worse with time. The incidence increases with age; about 50 percent of people over age eighty-five suffer some symptoms of dementia. Of this number, approximately 50 to 60 percent—about 4 million men and women over sixty-five—suffer from a type of dementia called Alzheimer's disease (AD), while another 20 percent have vascular dementia, in which a series of small strokes (brain attacks) damage or destroy brain tissue. In essence, vascular dementia is the result of clots or bleeding within the brain.

## What do scientists think is the connection between the B vitamins and Alzheimer's disease and other dementias?

As discussed in chapter 1, one of the main risk groups for B vitamin deficiencies are elder Americans who, for various reasons, fail to obtain all the vital nutrients they need to survive and thrive. Often, the first and most devastating symptoms of B vitamin deficiencies are those affecting the brain, causing dementia, anxiety, and depression. Here's why more and more experts believe that B vitamin deficiency could play a role in the development of Alzheimer's disease:

- *Vitamin $B_1$.* Because vitamin $B_1$ is essential for the synthesis and release of acetylcholine, the metabolism of the vitamin might be altered in Alzheimer's patients. A study conducted at the Medical College of Georgia, for instance, found that high doses of vitamin B (3 to 8 grams daily) slightly improved symptoms of dementia.

- *Vitamin $B_{12}$.* One of the functions of vitamin $B_{12}$ is to maintain healthy nerve tissue. A deficiency of the vitamin may contribute to the development and progression of the disease. Studies have shown that blood levels of vitamin $B_{12}$ are significantly lower in Alzheimer's patients than in patients suffering from other brain or memory disorders. Scores on cognitive function tests are lowest in Alzheimer patients with the lowest $B_{12}$ blood levels.

• *Choline*. The attempts to use this vitamin B–like substance are based on the observation that acetylcholine, which contains choline and is responsible for the transfer of messages related to memory, is not produced in sufficient amounts in the brains of patients with Alzheimer's disease. To date, however, studies have not shown a direct connection between increased intake of choline and improvement of Alzheimer's disease symptoms.

## What are the symptoms of AD?

No matter what acts as the initial trigger, as the disease progresses, memory, speech, and other aspects of cortical functioning begin to diminish. Usually, AD begins slowly, and the first symptoms are often simple forgetfulness: People with early-stage AD may have trouble recalling recent events, activities, or names of familiar people or things, and simple problems may become harder to solve. As the disease progresses, however, symptoms become more pronounced, prompting medical intervention. Routine tasks like dressing, bathing, and doing the dishes are forgotten. Talking, reading, and understanding become impossible. In addition, people with AD often suffer from anxiety, depression, and aggression.

**Are there any specific tests that can diagnose Alzheimer's disease?**

To date, no laboratory test exists that can diagnose Alzheimer's disease with any certainty. The only direct evidence is the presence of beta-amyloid plaques, which can only be viewed at autopsy after the patient's death. At specialized centers, however, experienced doctors are probably able to diagnose AD correctly 80 to 90 percent of the time. They do so first by ruling out any other possible causes of the patient's memory and cognitive problems through a thorough medical exam, which may include laboratory blood and urine tests as well as a brain scan.

**Is there treatment for Alzheimer's disease?**

At this time, no treatment exists that will cure Alzheimer's disease nor repair the damage done to the brain by cerebrovascular disease. Some medications may help improve symptoms and, perhaps, slow the progress of AD. However, without question, making sure that you receive all of the B vitamins necessary for the proper function of your brain and nervous system—throughout your life—may well go a long way in staving off the ravages of Alzheimer's disease and other diseases of the aging brain.

## DEPRESSION

At any age, depression is one of the most common health problems in the United States today. According to the National Institute of Mental Health, more than one in twenty Americans—some 17.8 million people—suffer from depression every year. Although there are many physical and personal circumstances that can lead to this potentially devastating disease, B vitamin deficiency can certainly be an important factor to consider, especially in the elderly.

It is important to recognize that depression is not merely a blue mood but a medical disorder that can affect your physical as well as your mental health. To give you an idea of how wide-ranging its effects can be, here is a list of common symptoms of depression:

- A persistent sad, anxious, or empty mood

- Sleeping too little or too much, or early awakening

- Reduced appetite and weight loss or increased appetite and weight gain

- Loss of interest and pleasure in activities once enjoyed

- Persistent physical symptoms—especially gastrointestinal problems, headaches, and pain—that don't respond to treatment

- Difficulty concentrating, remembering, or making decisions

- Fatigue or loss of energy

- Feelings of guilt and worthlessness

- Thoughts of death or suicide

Depression can be triggered both by emotional trauma and underlying psychological problems. It can also lead to or result from difficulties in coping with family, career, and personal challenges. Again, however, it's all too easy and common to ignore underlying malnutrition as the root cause, which is often a mistake when it comes to understanding and treating depression.

## Who is most at risk for depression?

Depression does not discriminate. The disorder affects people of every age, race, religion, and culture. It is neither an inevitable side effect of aging nor a disorder reserved for the young and stereotypically self-indulgent. In fact, each of us is more or less vulnerable to the disease, depending on a variety of factors. There appears to be a genetic component to depression, as people with a family history of the disease are at higher risk. Women tend to be more prone to depression than men, although new research indicates that men with depression may exhibit different symptoms such as aggression and substance abuse, and thus are misdiagnosed. Incidence of depression also increases with age, due probably in equal part to age-related physical changes in the body and brain and one's response to those changes. In addition, dealing with the loss of loved ones, coping with chronic illness, and losing one's independence also have an impact on mental and emotional health.

## How is depression treated medically?

In addition to psychotherapy to treat the underlying and resulting emotional challenges connected to depression, doctors now look toward drug therapy to treat this often stubborn disorder. In fact, prescriptions for antidepressants and stimulants by doctors increased dramatically from 1985 to 1994, according to a study published in the *Journal of the American Medical Association* on February 18, 1998. The number of visits during which a psychotropic medication was prescribed increased from 32.7 million to 45.6

million. Many of these drugs are highly effective in most people who take them, but they are not the answer for everyone.

One problem with the idea of solutions like Prozac and other forms of antidepressant medication is that they become quick fixes for both doctors and patients alike. Their ready availability may discourage doctors from looking for other potential causes of depression and other mental disorders, causes like underlying vitamin and mineral deficiencies. This is especially true because so few medical doctors, and perhaps even fewer psychotherapists, have a true understanding of nutrition and its relationship to mental health.

**My grandmother seems depressed and out of sorts. Could taking supplements of B-complex vitamins help her?**

There's every indication that it would help. Supplementation with one or more of the vitamin Bs may be especially helpful for the elderly who are depressed or cognitively impaired, since they generally are at much higher risk of running vitamin B deficiencies. A study published in the *Journal of the American College of Nutrition* (11, 1992: 159–163), for instance, showed that after just four weeks of treatment with 10 milligrams each of $B_1$, $B_2$, and $B_6$ (about five to eight times the RDI) patients experienced improved status on cognitive function testing.

**I've been taking Prozac, but it hasn't been working. Will B vitamins help?**

A recent review of a series of studies indicates that it just might. A study in a 1997 issue of *Nutrition Review* found that people who don't respond well to Prozac and other antidepressants that work by improving the way brain cells use serotonin (called selective serotonin reuptake inhibitors) are also deficient in folic acid. Research continues to focus on the connection between the two. In any case, boosting your B vitamin intake would have many benefits to your body, mind, and soul, so as long as you talk to your doctor beforehand, you might want to experiment to see if taking more folic acid also alleviates your depressive symptoms.

So far, you've read about the way the B vitamins affect several vital body systems and processes, including the healthy growth of a fetus, the cardiovascular system, the development of cancer, and the vitality of the brain and the nervous system. But the effects of B vitamins are felt in almost every part of the body, as you'll see in the next chapter, in which we take you from head to toe to show you the healing properties and the preventive potential of these remarkable nutrients.

## REFERENCES FOR CHAPTER SEVEN

Alpert, JE; Fava, M. "Nutrition and depression: the role of folate." *Nutrition Review*, 1997; 55 (5): 145–149.

Fava, M; Borus, JS; Alpert, JE; et al. "Folate, vitamin $B_{12}$, and homocysteine in major depressive disorder." *American Journal of Psychiatry*, 1997; 154 (3): 426–428.

Gelenberg. AJ; Wojcik, JD; et al. "Tyrosine for the treatment of depression." *American Journal of Psychiatry*, 1980; 137: 622–623.

Hasanah, CI; Khan, UA; et al. "Reduced red-cell folate in mania." *Journal of Affective Disorders*, 1997; 46 (2): 95–99.

Holmes, JM. "Cerebral manifestations of vitamin $B_{12}$ deficiency." *Journal of Nutritional Medicine*, 1991; 2: 89–90.

Hutto, BR. "Folate and cobalamin in psychiatric illness." *Comprehensive Psychiatry,* 1997; 38 (6): 304–314.

Langlais PJ. "Alcohol-related thiamin deficiency." *Alcohol Health and Research World*, 1955; 19 (2): 113–121.

Martinson, EW. "Benefits of exercise for the treatment of depression." *Sports Medicine*, 1990; 9: 380–389.

Reynolds, E.; et al. "Folate deficiency in depressive illness." *British Journal of Psychiatry*, 1970; 117: 287–292.

Zheng, JJ; Rosenberg, IH. "What is the nutritional status of the elderly?" *Geriatrics*, 1989; 44 (6): 57–58.

# · 8 ·

# A Head-to-Toe, A-to-Z Guide to
# Your Health and the Bs

In this chapter we take you on a tour of the illnesses and conditions that the B vitamins are known to help alleviate. In some cases, the ties are direct and very well documented. In other cases, the evidence is more anecdotal. Either way, you know that by taking at least the RDIs for the B vitamins, you'll be promoting health and vitality in every cell of your body, especially if you're already feeling ill and under the weather. Furthermore, and this is an important fact to keep in mind, if you're taking medication for any condition—particularly if you're taking antibiotics—you should boost your intake of B vitamins because the medication could be depleting your stores of these nutrients.

In the meantime, let's explore how one or more of the B vitamins might help alleviate a minor or more serious condition that's holding you back from enjoying life to its fullest.

## ACNE

Acne is a general term for a variety of skin conditions involving inflammation of the oil-producing glands of the skin. The most common type of acne is called acne vulgaris, and it usually strikes in the teenage years and continues through the twenties. Women in particular tend to suffer from this condition in later years, probably because of the hormone imbalances that occur from time to time. Psychological stress may also trigger acne flare-ups.

Medical treatment for acne ranges from hormonal treatments in the form of birth control pills for women, and prescription drugs such as Accutane, which contains a powerful derivative of vitamin A.

### THE ROLE OF THE Bs

Evidence suggests that the B vitamins help alleviate acne, especially in women. Taking supplements can help in two ways: First, as you know, the B vitamins are important in maintaining the health of the skin in general. Riboflavin, pantothenic acid, and $B_6$ are especially known for their abilities to reduce facial oiliness and blackhead formation. Second, B vitamins help regulate the production of sex hormones like estrogen; without enough of the Bs, hormonal imbalances may occur that trigger acne flare-ups.

■ **Vitamin B Prescription**
Vitamin B complex containing 400 micrograms folic acid and 25 milligrams per day of the other B vitamins. Extra vitamin $B_6$ 25 milligrams per day, especially for acne aggravated by menstrual cycles or menopause.

## OTHER HELPFUL NUTRITIONAL HINTS

Eating a healthy, balanced diet will help keep all body systems—including those that maintain the skin—up and running. Regular exercise will help bring oxygen and nutrients to the cells of the skin and, more importantly, facilitate the removal of waste products such as bacteria from these tissues.

As for other supplements, vitamin A is especially beneficial for clear, healthy skin, and some doctors recommend using supplements of about 5,000 to 10,000 IU daily. Taking vitamin A in the form of beta-carotene is also recommended. Zinc, in doses of 15 to 30 milligrams, helps to suppress bacterial infections and maintain the health of the oil-producing glands of the skin.

## ALLERGIES

About one in every five Americans—roughly 46 million men, women, and children—suffer from allergies, a syndrome of diseases that involves a sensitivity to a substance that is ordinarily harmless. An allergy occurs when the body's defense system, called the immune system, does not work properly. In effect, the immune system treats a substance like pollen as a deadly enemy that must be eliminated at all costs. The symptoms of an allergy—watery eyes, wheezing, swelling, itchy skin, etc.—represent the body's efforts to rid itself of the offending substance.

Susceptibility to an allergen (a substance that triggers a reaction) depends on a variety of factors, including heredity and general state of health. Stress, poor diet, and infections can set the stage for allergic reactions to occur and certainly exacerbate them when they do.

Medical treatment of less severe allergies consists of the use of antihistamines and decongestants. Antihistamines are drugs that reduce the action of histamines, body chemicals involved in the allergic response that cause the majority of allergic symptoms. Decongestants help clear the stuffiness of the nasal passages that often occur with allergies. For more severe allergies, doctors prescribe corticosteroids, powerful anti-inflammatory drugs, and cromolyn sodium, a nonsteroidal medication for respiratory allergies. All of these drugs have serious side effects, especially over the long term.

## THE ROLE OF THE BS

Vitamins $B_1$, $B_3$, and $B_6$ are particularly helpful in reducing anxiety, which can help alleviate the cycle of frustration and discomfort many people with allergies endure. In addition, because the B vitamins are so crucial in the manufacture of certain immune system cells, a deficit of these nutrients could create an imbalance that might lead to an overreaction of the whole system.

### ▪ Vitamin B Prescription
Vitamin B complex 10 milligrams three times per day. Pantothenic acid 250 to 500 milligrams three times a day.

## OTHER HELPFUL NUTRITIONAL HINTS

Taking other vitamin and mineral antioxidants such as vitamins C, E, beta-carotene, and selenium can help reduce the damage that free radical cells do to the tissues of the body. Even if antioxidants don't directly help solve the allergic problem, they will help your body remain strong against other infections that may attack when you're trying to fight against the harmless allergens. Quercitin and other bioflavonoids have natural antihistamine activity.

## ARTHRITIS AND GOUT

In the United States today, more than 15 percent of the population—about 40 million people—suffer from arthritis. This disease, of which there are more than 100 different forms, involves the inflammation of joints, surrounding tendons, ligaments, and cartilage, as well as destruction of bone. It can affect any part of the body, from the feet to the knees, back, shoulders, elbows, and, in certain types of arthritis, the heart, lungs, and other organs. There are two main types of arthritis: osteoarthritis, which primarily affects older people and involves a wearing down of the cartilage and bones in various joints; and rheumatoid arthritis, which is a systemic disease involving an inflammatory process in the joints and, often, in several organ systems as well.

In addition, gout is a related disease in which tiny crystals form in the joint space when the level of certain blood chemicals becomes too high. White blood cells rush to the site, causing the joint to become inflamed and painful. Gout occurs when too much uric acid, a blood protein, is present in the body.

Medical treatment of arthritis usually involves an exercise program designed to keep the joints as flexible—and the muscles that support them as strong—as possible. If the disease is mild, the use of heating pads and hot baths may help the joints become more limber and loose, as does the use of aspirin and other anti-inflammatory drugs. With more severe cases of rheumatoid arthritis, a drug called methotrexate is often used. This medication, while useful in limiting the inflammatory process, can be toxic to the body, as can many other medications used to treat chronic arthritis.

## THE ROLE OF B VITAMINS

All of the B vitamins are considered important to the development and maintenance of bones and muscle, and thus essential to the health of one's joints. In addition, vitamins $B_1$, $B_3$, and $B_6$ are particularly helpful in reducing anxiety, which can help alleviate the cycle of pain that many people with arthritis must endure. Pantothenic acid is a component in the manufacture of cartilage. In addition, it is essential in the production of steroid hormones, necessary to keep the immune system up and running during times of physical stress. A form of vitamin $B_3$ known as niacinamide seems to have a positive effect on arthritis as well, especially in high doses of 250 milligrams every few hours. (Since niacinamide may affect the liver, however, talk to your doctor before taking high doses of this vitamin.) Finally, several recent studies show that using folic acid along with the anti-arthritis medication methotrexate helps reduce the drug's toxicity. Thus, many doctors are prescribing folic acid along with methotrexate to their arthritis patients.

### ■ Vitamin B Prescription

A dose of 25 to 100 milligrams of vitamin B complex, preferably in a timed-release form, may help alleviate symptoms of both types of arthritis. Taking an extra dose of vitamin $B_6$, of up to 50 milligrams per day, may also be helpful. Folic acid 800 micrograms twice daily can be helpful in lessening gouty arthritis.

## OTHER HELPFUL NUTRITIONAL HINTS

A multivitamin-mineral supplement that contains 100 percent of the RDI for all essential nutrients combined with regular exercise and a healthy diet can go a long way in treating the symptoms of arthritis. Furthermore, boosting your intake of antioxidants can help prevent more damage to the cells of the muscles that free radicals can cause.

Some minerals are especially important when it comes to the health of the bones, muscles, and joints. Calcium and magnesium, taken in conjunction with one another, help maintain the integrity of the bones. Glucosamine, now available in supplement form, is a naturally occurring substance found in high concentrations in joint structure. It appears that this chemical plays an integral part in stimulating the production of connective tissue and new cartilage growth so that the body can repair the damage done to these structures by arthritis. The standard dose for glucosamine sulfate supplements is about 500 milligrams three times a day.

When it comes to gout, nutrition is extremely important. Among the nutritional guidelines to follow are: avoiding alcohol, maintaining a proper weight, and avoiding foods that contain purines, which are chemicals that can raise the levels of uric acid and thus precipitate an attack of gout. Purines are found in organ meats, sardines, and anchovies.

## ASTHMA

Asthma is a chronic respiratory condition most often related to allergies. Attacks of asthma may be related to contact with an allergen or may be precipitated by physical or emotional stress. Symptoms of asthma include difficulty breathing, wheezing, and tightness in the chest. Violent coughing often occurs. An asthma attack can last from a few minutes to several days.

Medical treatment for asthma includes many of the same medications used to treat allergies, namely corticosteroids and antihistamines. In addition, a mainstay of asthma treatment are bronchodilators, drugs that act to open up constricted breathing passages in the lungs.

## THE ROLE OF THE BS

All of the B complex vitamins help reduce anxiety and stress, which frequently precipitate an attack as well as prolong and exacerbate attacks when they do occur. In particular, increased intake of vitamin $B_6$ might help reduce the symptoms of asthma, as some studies show that asthma patients have lower blood levels of vitamin $B_6$ than do healthy adults. Vitamin $B_{12}$ is known to prevent and treat respiratory allergies as well.

### ■ Vitamin B Prescription
Vitamin B complex 25 milligrams with extra vitamin $B_6$ 25 milligrams two times per day. Sublingual $B_{12}$ 100 micrograms per day.

## OTHER HELPFUL NUTRITIONAL HINTS

As is true for the allergies that may accompany asthma, it is important to pinpoint—if possible—the triggers of asthma and—again, if possible—to avoid them in the future. In addition, you may want to increase your intake of vitamin A, which is necessary for the general health of the lungs, and vitamin E, which as a powerful antioxidant helps protect against airborne allergens. Fish oils or flaxseed oil are also helpful.

## BALDNESS

Hair loss occurs for a variety of reasons. Many forms of hair loss are genetic in origin; male pattern baldness, for instance, comprises about 90 percent of hair loss cases and is known to run in families. Hormonal factors, aging, stress, certain medications, and several different diseases can also cause hair loss in both men and women. One of the most common causes of nonhereditary cases of hair loss is poor eating habits that result in vitamin and mineral deficiencies, especially crash dieting.

In recent decades, new medical treatments have become available for some cases of hair loss. Rogaine is a prescription drug that contains a substance called minoxidil that appears to stimulate hair growth in some people.

### THE ROLE OF THE BS

The B vitamins help alleviate stress, which is a contributing factor in many cases of hair loss. Evidence suggests that pantothenic acid has the power to help regenerate and restore shine and color to the hair, and biotin appears to enhance hair growth, thicken fibers, and diminish shedding. Taking extra biotin and pantothenic acid along with a high-potency multivitamin and/or B-complex supplement will help keep your hair as healthy as possible, no matter how genetics affects your pattern of growth and loss.

▪ **Vitamin B Prescription**
Vitamin B complex with 50 micrograms $B_{12}$, 50 micrograms biotin, 400 micrograms folic acid, and 50 milligrams of other B vitamins. Take twice daily.

## OTHER HELPFUL NUTRITIONAL HINTS

In addition to making sure you get enough of the Bs, looking at your iron intake is the next most important element in your diet when it comes to the health of your hair—at least when it comes to hair loss in women. (For men, genetics accounts for much more of the equation.) Along with the iron, it's important to also increase your intake of vitamin C, which helps your body absorb and use iron more efficiently.

# CARPAL TUNNEL SYNDROME

Carpal tunnel syndrome is a painful orthopedic condition that affects the hands and wrists. The carpal tunnel is a passageway through the wrist (carpal is from the Greek word *karpalis*, which means wrist) that is bounded by bones and ligaments. It protects the nerves and tendons that extend into the hand. When the tissue that forms the carpal tunnel becomes swollen and inflamed, the condition compresses the median nerve—the nerve that provides sensation to the thumb, index, middle, and ring fingers. Pressure on this nerve leads to numbness and pain. Carpal tunnel syndrome most often develops in people who use repetitive motions in their work or home life. Word processors, carpenters, grocery clerks, and violinists are among those who are frequent sufferers of this syndrome.

Medical treatment for carpal tunnels includes simply

resting the joint for a period of weeks or months and wearing a splint that immobilizes the wrists but allows the hand to function almost normally. Medication in the form of a corticosteroid, such as cortisone, may help alleviate the pain, but doctors don't usually prescribe it unless the more conservative approach of rest and recovery fails. If the pain is persistent, surgery to divide the ligament that presses on the nerve may be suggested.

## THE ROLE OF THE Bs

Because vitamin $B_6$ is so crucial in the development and maintenance of healthy nerve tissue, a deficiency of the nutrient may contribute to the development or exacerbation of the syndrome. In fact, studies show that people who suffer from carpal tunnel syndrome tend to have vitamin $B_6$ deficiencies. Many practitioners use a combination of vitamin $B_6$, $B_2$, and $B_3$ to treat this disorder.

### ▪ Vitamin B Prescription

Vitamin B complex 25 milligrams with extra vitamin $B_6$ 25 milligrams three times per day for two months, then two times per day.

## THE ROLE OF OTHER NUTRIENTS

Magnesium 200 to 400 milligrams per day should be taken along with the extra $B_6$.

Regular exercise—of the entire body as well as exercises that focus on strengthening and stretching the arm, wrist, hand, and fingers—will help both prevent the disease from occurring and treating its symptoms. Consuming a diet high in fiber, vitamins, and minerals and low in fat, sugar, and processed foods will help maintain health in all body systems, including the muscles, joints, and nerves involved in carpal tunnel syndrome.

# ECZEMA AND DERMATITIS

Eczema and dermatitis are general terms for any chronic skin inflammation or irritation. Symptoms include dryness, scaling, and oozing of the skin. Eczema and dermatitis often develop from allergic reactions to any one of a number of substances, including but not limited to pollen, dust, pet dander, or chemical irritants. Many cases of these skin disorders can be traced to food allergies. Stress, lack of sleep, and anxiety can exacerbate the condition.

## THE ROLE OF THE BS

Because the B vitamins are involved in the maintenance of the skin, it should come as no surprise that a deficiency of any one or more of these vitamins could produce symptoms of eczema and dermatitis. That's especially true for niacin and $B_6$ deficiencies in which skin disorders are usually the first and most common results. Making sure that you get at least the RDIs of all of the B vitamins, along with extra niacin (make sure you talk to your doctor first) and $B_6$ may help alleviate the problem. Doing so will also help you manage stress better, which can help break the cycle of tension, stress, and dermatitis outbreaks.

### ▪ Vitamin B Prescription
Vitamin B complex 25 milligrams two times per day. You may try an extra niacin 250 milligrams two times per day, with your doctor's knowledge.

## OTHER HELPFUL NUTRITIONAL HINTS

As is true for allergies, the first line of defense against the development of eczema and dermatitis is the identification and elimination of its triggers. Making sure that you eat a balanced, healthy diet that limits the intake of sugar and processed flour may also help. Some people find that tomatoes and citrus fruits are particularly troublesome; others find that eating certain dairy products and processed foods trigger outbreaks. Taking extra vitamin C may help reduce the inflammation associated with these skin conditions. Vitamin A is also essential for maintaining healthy skin tissue.

## EYESTRAIN AND VISION PROBLEMS

The gift of vision is one of our most precious, but there are few among us who take the time to consider what our eyes need in the way of nutrition to stay healthy and vital. Nutritional deficiencies can trigger or exacerbate minor conditions, such as itching and dimness of sight (called amblyopia), as well as more serious conditions like cataracts, glaucoma, and age-related macular degeneration.

Cataracts are a major cause of vision loss worldwide, affecting more than 20 million people. A cataract is a clouding of the normally clear lens of the eye. The clouding of the lens—which is one of the two main focusing mechanisms of the eye—blocks the passage of light needed for sight. Almost everyone develops some clouding in the eye lenses with aging, but age is not the only factor in the development of the condition. Certain diseases, including diabetes, can contribute to the formation of cataracts, as can severe nutritional deficiencies. Treatment of cataracts may include the use of prescription eyedrops that widen the pupil to bring in more light. In most cases, surgery to remove the cataract is quite successful.

Glaucoma is the leading cause of blindness in the United States, affecting about 2 million people mostly over the age of sixty-five. The disease involves a buildup of pressure in the space between the lens and the cornea of the eye, usually because something prevents proper drainage of liquid from this area. This pressure affects the fibers of the optic nerve, slowly damaging them and resulting in loss of vision.

Age-related macular degeneration occurs when small deposits form and blood vessels grow in the central portion of the retina, the main focusing part of the eye. If these vessels leak, the retinal cells responsible for central vision are damaged. Eventually, a scar may develop, producing considerable vision loss. The only treatment for macular degeneration is laser therapy to seal the leaky blood vessels.

## THE ROLE OF THE B VITAMINS

Acting as both antioxidants and cell membrane protectors, the B vitamins help to maintain healthy vision throughout the life cycle. In addition, their roles in synthesizing DNA help keep the cells of the eyes regenerating at a normal rate. A deficiency of these vitamins can lead to such symptoms as itchiness, burning, and temporary lack of focus. This is especially true when it comes to vitamin $B_2$: One of the hallmark symptoms of moderate to severe vitamin $B_2$ deficiency is burning and itching of the eyes. The outer lining of the eyes becomes inflamed, and ulcers may appear on the cornea. In addition, low vitamin B intake is also associated with cataract formation; more than 80 percent of people with cataracts also have low levels of serum $B_2$. A recent study at the National Cancer Institute and National Eyes Institute reports that supplements of vitamin $B_2$ delay cataract formation in the elderly.

### ▪ Vitamin B Prescription
Vitamin B complex containing riboflavin 25 milligrams two times per day.

## OTHER HELPFUL NUTRITIONAL HINTS

Antioxidants such as vitamins A, C, and E have long been known to help protect against and to improve vision problems. Intake of sufficient vitamin A has been associated with a decreased risk of both cataracts and macular degeneration. As for vitamin E, a 1991 study of 350 men and women found that people who took daily supplements of more than 400 IU of vitamin E had less than half the risk of developing cataracts than did people who took no supplements.

Another nutrient important for vision is zinc. Like the B vitamins, zinc helps to synthesize the nucleic acids RNA and DNA, which are essential for cell division, cell repair, and growth. Zinc is found in the iris and retina and may be involved in the activation of vitamin A. Selenium is another mineral that protects the eye.

Finally, substances called omega-3 fatty acids, which are found in fish oils, also help to maintain eyesight. Large amounts of these fats are found in eye tissue, and a deficiency of them may affect vision, at least during early childhood development.

# FATIGUE

Perhaps the most common complaint of modern Americans is fatigue, the feeling of general weakness, lethargy, and apathy. There are many causes of fatigue, some related to other illnesses, most stemming from lack of exercise and poor nutrition. Indeed, even a marginal deficiency of any nutrient can lead to feelings of fatigue. In addition to general malaise, there appears to be a separate syndrome, called chronic fatigue syndrome (CFS), that some scientists believe is caused by the Epstein-Barr virus, the same virus that causes infectious mononucleosis in teenagers. In addition to feelings of weakness and exhaustion, CFS causes headache, sore throat, swollen lymph nodes, backache, irritability, and indigestion.

## THE ROLE OF THE BS

Anemia—the lack of sufficient red blood cells that carry oxygen to the tissues of the body—is one of the most common causes of fatigue, and a deficiency of the B vitamins can trigger this condition. In addition, many of the B vitamins, including vitamin $B_1$, vitamin $B_2$, vitamin $B_6$, pantothenic acid, and niacin are essential for converting food into energy. Thus, a deficiency of one or more of these vitamins can lead to fatigue and decreased energy.

### ▪ Vitamin B Prescription
Vitamin B complex with 50 micrograms $B_{12}$, 50 milligrams biotin, 400 micrograms folic acid, and 50 milligrams of other B vitamins. Take twice daily.

## OTHER HELPFUL NUTRITIONAL HINTS

Needless to say, in order to feel well-rested and vital, eating a balanced diet and getting plenty of regular exercise are absolute necessities. Exercise is especially important because it helps release endorphins, body chemicals that act to relieve both physical and emotional pain. Bolstering your intake of vitamin C and other antioxidants can help boost your immune system and protect you against infection, which certainly can wear you down. Minerals, particularly magnesium and potassium, are important in generating energy. Iron deficiency can cause fatigue as well as anemia. Drinking plenty of water—sixty-four ounces of it or more every day—can help keep your system flushed of impurities and waste and thus more efficient.

## GINGIVITIS AND OTHER GUM PROBLEMS

The cells that line the mouth have a short life span and require a constant supply of nutrients for normal repair, replacement, and maintenance of these tissues. Gum disease begins with excess plaque, a material made of a mixture of food, bacteria, and mucus that attaches to the teeth and the gums. If not removed, plaque becomes calculus, a hard substance that irritates and infects the gums. This leads to a disease called gingivitis, which is characterized by red, swollen, and bleeding gums. If left untreated, gingivitis can progress to become pyorrhea, which involves inflammation of the gums, gum recession, and loss of teeth.

Interestingly, new evidence points to a connection between gum disease and heart disease. It appears that the bacteria that invade the gums with gingivitis may enter the bloodstream and affect the heart. Studies show, for instance, that patients who see their dentist at least once a year for cleaning have a risk of stroke four times smaller than patients who don't see a dentist on a regular basis. In addition, investigators continue to explore whether homocysteine—the body chemical now implicated as a serious risk factor for heart disease and which is related to low folic acid and other B vitamin levels—may be implicated in gingivitis and other gum diseases.

## THE ROLE OF THE B VITAMINS

Scientists have long been aware that the B vitamins—particularly $B_2$—play important roles in the health of the gums and teeth. In fact, early symptoms of vitamin $B_2$ deficiency include burning and soreness of the mouth, lips, and tongue, and the lining of the mouth becomes inflamed in advanced stages of vitamin $B_2$ deficiency. Vitamin $B_{12}$ and folic acid are also important, mainly because they help to maintain and repair the cells of the gums.

### ▪ Vitamin B Prescription

Vitamin B complex containing riboflavin 25 milligrams, 50 micrograms of $B_{12}$, 400 micrograms folic acid. Take twice daily. Also, get liquid folic acid, dip a cotton swab in the folic acid and swab the gum line nightly, followed by gentle brushing.

## OTHER HELPFUL NUTRITIONAL HINTS

Proper hygiene in the form of regular brushing, flossing, and visits to the dentist are the mainstay of gum and tooth health. Eating lots of crunchy fresh fruit and vegetables will help scrape plaque from the teeth and provide the body with antioxidants that will protect against infection all at the same time. Drinking vitamin D–fortified milk helps provide the raw materials your body needs to maintain the health of the teeth. A number of different vitamins and minerals can help as well, including vitamin A (important in tooth formation), vitamin D (which helps regulate the growth of teeth by its interactions with the minerals calcium and phosphorus), vitamin C (required for the normal formation of the connective tissue that holds together the gums and other tissues), calcium (which strengthens the jawbone and the teeth), magnesium (which works with calcium to form and maintain healthy teeth and bones), and zinc (which along with vitamin C and folic acid helps to form healthy gum tissue as well as to protect against bacterial infection).

## INFLAMMATORY BOWEL DISEASE

These two conditions—ulcerative colitis and Crohn's disease—together represent the conditions called inflammatory bowel disease. The conditions are similar in symptoms and in their general causes: Both are chronic conditions in which an inflammatory reaction, characterized by tiny ulcers and small abscesses, affects the digestive tract. While Crohn's disease can involve any portion of the intestinal tract, ulcerative colitis is confined to the colon. Symptoms include abdominal pain, diarrhea, and constipation, which can result in weight loss, dehydration, and anemia. No one knows what causes inflammatory bowel disease, but heredity plays a role in some cases. Depression, stress, and anxiety may trigger or exacerbate the conditions.

Treatment of inflammatory bowel disease usually consists of corticosteroid medication, often in the form of enemas that bring relief to the tissues of the colon and large intestine. In addition to alleviating the inflammatory process, treatment focuses on replacing the nutrients lost to the disease through severe diarrhea, which usually requires vitamin and mineral supplements. Approximately 20 to 25 percent of those with inflammatory bowel disease will require surgery at some time to remove portions of the damaged colon or rectum.

## THE ROLE OF THE B VITAMINS

Because of the important role that the B vitamins play in the metabolism of proteins and carbohydrates, replacing them should they become deficient—as they so often do in this disease—is of utmost importance. Unfortunately, many people with this condition find it difficult to digest dairy products and cruciferous vegetables (like the folic acid–rich broccoli and cabbage). If you suffer from inflammatory bowel disease, it's more important than ever to bolster your daily intake of the B vitamins and other nutrients by taking high-potency supplements. In particularly severe cases, $B_6$ along with magnesium is given by injection to relax the muscles and control the colon.

### ■ Vitamin B Prescription
Vitamin B complex with 50 micrograms $B_{12}$, 50 micrograms biotin, 400 micrograms folic acid, and 50 milligrams of other B vitamins. Take three times daily. Extra PABA 500 milligrams three times per day can also be used in acute flare-ups.

## OTHER HELPFUL NUTRITIONAL HINTS

Studies suggest that fish oils can lessen the inflammation of IBD. Zinc and vitamin E are also helpful.

Most doctors recommend that their patients with colitis or Crohn's disease consume five or six small meals rather than two or three large ones per day to aid in digestion. It is also important to limit the intake of saturated fats (such as butter and vegetable oil), as these substances can encourage inflammation and diarrhea. Adding foods high in roughage that do not irritate the digestive tract is important; brown rice and other grain brans can help soothe while adding bulk.

## OSTEOPOROSIS

Osteoporosis, or bone loss, affects at least half of all American women over the age of sixty. Osteoporosis is a long process of bone degeneration that may start as early as thirty to forty years before the first signs appear. The term osteoporosis comes from the Greek *osteo* meaning bone and *porus* meaning pore or passage. With osteoporosis, your bones become too weak to support the body. It occurs because your bones do not receive adequate nourishment to grow and renew themselves, nor are they able to efficiently metabolize the nutrients they do receive. Recent evidence exists to suggest that high levels of homocysteine may be involved in the osteoporotic process, perhaps by restricting blood flow to the bones.

Among the risk factors for the development of osteoporosis are the following:

- *Gender.* According to the National Osteoporosis Foundation, women are four times more likely than men to develop osteoporosis. Experts believe that the same mechanism that protects women from heart disease at a younger age also protects them from osteoporosis.

- *Age.* The older you are, the thinner your bones will probably be, largely because the cells of the body regenerate less efficiently the older you are—perhaps because of your nutritional status.

- *Heredity.* Women with a family history of osteoporosis are more likely to develop the disease.

- *Physical build.* Because petite women with small bone structures have less bone mass to start with, they are at a much higher risk of osteoporosis.

- *Lifestyle.* Cigarette smoking, sedentary lifestyle, excess intake of alcohol and caffeine, and the failure to eat a healthy, balanced diet or take supplements to meet at least the minimal RDIs for all the vitamins and minerals puts a woman at increased risk. So, too, does taking certain prescription medications, particularly corticosteroids, antibiotics, and diuretics to treat high blood pressure.

Prevention is the very best medicine when it comes to osteoporosis, so making sure you meet your daily requirements of important vitamins and minerals and exercising on a regular basis will help you avoid this disease at a later age. Treatment of osteoporosis once it occurs involves obtaining plenty of calcium and magnesium, either from the diet or in supplement form, getting as much exercise as possible under a doctor's supervision. Certain medications may also help prevent further bone loss and may even help restore some strength. These include estrogen replacement therapy for women after menopause and two bone-sparing drugs called etidronate and calcitonine.

## THE ROLE OF THE Bs

Because of their role in the growth and maintenance of cell membranes, including bone and blood cells, the B vitamins are especially helpful in preventing the onset of osteoporosis. Furthermore, because folic acid, vitamin $B_6$, and vitamin $B_{12}$ are especially important in reducing levels of homocysteine, they may also protect against the ravages this toxic chemical may do to bone tissue.

▪ **Vitamin B Prescription**
Vitamin B complex 25 milligrams two times per day.

## OTHER HELPFUL NUTRITIONAL HINTS

Exercise is vitally important for bone health, especially weight-bearing exercise (running, walking, and weight training) that helps build bones and the muscles that support them. A healthy diet, rich in vitamins and minerals, is also important. Dairy products—skim milk, yogurt, and cheese—help provide enough vitamin D, calcium, and magnesium, and those who are lactose intolerant can get those nutrients by eating plenty of spinach, broccoli, bok choy, and figs.

# PREMENSTRUAL SYNDROME

According to the Premenstrual Institute, up to 40 percent of women of childbearing age suffer from some degree of premenstrual syndrome. Sometimes PMS begins with the first menstruation, but sometimes it doesn't appear until after a woman has given birth for the first time or is experiencing a period of major stress. PMS may be hereditary and may become worse with age as hormonal fluctuations become more marked. Doctors are still unsure of the exact cause of PMS in individual women but are now convinced that the syndrome does exist and does cause serious, sometimes disabling symptoms.

Symptoms may be both physical and emotional. Physical symptoms include bloating, swollen/painful breasts, swollen hands and feet, weight gain, food cravings, headaches, skin problems, and dizziness. Emotional problems may involve short temper, aggression, anger, anxiety/panic, confusion, depression, and lack of concentration.

Treatment of PMS may involve taking anti-inflammatory drugs such as ibuprofen or, for some women, taking birth control pills to control the hormonal swings that may lead to many PMS syndromes. In more severe and chronic cases, the use of antidepressants may be indicated.

## THE ROLE OF THE Bs

Because vitamin $B_6$ is a necessary nutrient in the manufacture of neurotransmitters—including serotonin, which helps regulate mood—a deficiency of vitamin $B_6$ may trigger some of the psychological symptoms of PMS. Ironically, some scientists believe that the fluctuations of estrogen and other hormones may deplete the body's supply of $B_6$, which only exacerbates the problem. Vitamin $B_6$ may also reduce breast pain and tenderness. Much research remains to be done in this area, but many women find that increasing their intake of $B_6$, along with taking a high-potency multivitamin and/or B-complex supplement, alleviates their symptoms every month.

■ **Vitamin B Prescription**

Vitamin B complex 25 milligrams with extra vitamin $B_6$ 25 milligrams two times per day.

## OTHER HELPFUL NUTRITIONAL HINTS

Many women find that certain foods trigger PMS symptoms, including sugar, caffeine, salt, and alcohol. In fact, a study published in a 1982 issue of the *Journal of Applied Nutrition* examined the dietary patterns of thirty-nine women with PMS compared with fourteen women who did not suffer from the symptoms. Those with PMS all consumed more refined sugar, refined carbohydrates, and dairy products than did those without the problem. Healthy women consumed considerably more—up to 45 percent more—B vitamins, iron, zinc, and manganese.

## REFERENCES FOR CHAPTER EIGHT

Akata, T; Sekiguchi, S; Takahashi, M; et al. "Successful combined treatment with vitamin $B_{12}$ and bright artificial light of one case with delayed sleep phase syndrome." *Japanese Journal of Psychiatric Neurology*, 1993; 47: 439–440.

Bernstein, A. "Vitamin $B_6$ in clinical neurology." *Annals of the New York Academy of Sciences*, 1990; 585: 250–260.

Brautbar, N; Gruber, H. "Magnesium and bone disease." *Nephron*, 1986; 44: 1–7.

Copeland, D; Stoukides, C. "Pyroxidine in carpal tunnel syndrome." *Annals of Pharmacology*, 1994; 28 (9): 1042–1044.

DeStafano, F; Anda, RF; Kahn, HS, et al. "Dental disease and risk of coronary heart mortality." *British Medical Journal*, 1993; 306 (6879): 688–691.

# Index

Acetyl coenzyme, 40
Acetylcholine, 30, 40, 133, 135
Acne, 150–151
Acute myocardial infarctions (heart
    attacks), 101–102
AD (Alzheimer's disease), 140–143
Additives, 71
Aerobic exercise (cardiovascular
    fitness), 64
AFP (alpha-fetoprotein) test, 82
Age
    cancer factor, 120
    cardiovascular disease factor, 96
Alcohol
    nervous system and, 136–140
    pregnancy and, 85
    vitamin deficiencies from, 6–7,
        19, 32, 85, 137–140
*All About B Vitamins* (Berkson), 42
Allergies, 151–153
Alpha-fetoprotein (AFP) test, 82
Alzheimer's disease (AD), 140–143
American Cancer Society, 121
American Heart Association, 13, 97,
    99, 103, 110, 111
*American Journal of Clinical
    Nutrition*, 68
American Lung Association, 110

Amygdala, 134
Anaerobic exercise (strength
    training), 64
Androgens, 118
Anencephaly, 82
Angina (chest pain), 102
*Annals of Internal Medicine*, 15
Antibiotics, 19
Antioxidants. *See also* Beta-
    carotene; Free radicals;
    Vitamin A; Vitamin C;
    Vitamin E
    for allergies, 152–153
    for cancer, 116, 117
    for cardiovascular disease, 108–
        109
    defined, 11, 12–13
    selenium, for allergies, 152
Aorta, 93
Appetite and vitamins, 7, 18–19.
    *See also* Diet and nutrition
Arteries, 93–94
Arteriosclerosis, 95, 97, 98, 99,
    102, 103
Arthritis and gout, 39, 153–155
Asthma, 39, 155–157
Atherosclerosis, 94
Axons, 132, 133